World Federation of Neurology
Seminars in Clinical Neurology

DYSTONIA

World Federation of Neurology
Seminars in Clinical Neurology

Dystonia

FACULTY
Joseph Jankovic, M.D., CHAIR
Professor of Neurology
Director of Parkinson's Disease Center and Movement Disorders Clinic
Department of Neurology, Baylor College of Medicine
Houston, Texas

Cynthia A. Comella, MD
Chair, Department of Neurology,
Beth Israel Medical Center
Professor, Department of Neurology,
Albert Einstien College of Medicine
New York, New York

Susan B. Bressman, MD
Neurological Institute,
Columbia Presbyterian Medical Center
New York, New York

Michele Tagliati, MD
Associate Professor
Division Chief, Movement Disorders
Mount Sinai School of Medicine
New York, New York

Michael Pourfar, MD
Division of Movement Disorders
Fellow, Department of Neurology
Columbia University Medical Center
New York, New York

Joseph K.C. Tsui, MBBS, MRCP, F.R CP(C)
Department of Neurology,
University of British Columbia
Vancouver, British Columbia, Canada

Mark A. Stacy, MD
Medical Director, Division of Neurology,
Duke University
Durham, North Carolina

M. Fiorella Contarino, MD
Istituto di Neuroligia,
Universit Cattolica
Roma, Italy

Alberto Albanese, MD
Istituto Nazionale Neurologica Carol Besta
Milano, Italy

Daniel Truong, MD
The Parkinson's and Movement
Disorders Institute
Fountain Valley, California

Mayank Pathak, MD
The Parkinson's and Movement
Disorders Institute
Fountain Valley, California

Karen Frei, MD
The Parkinson's and Movement
Disorders Institute
Fountain Valley, California

Series Editor
Theodore L. Munsat, MD
Professor of Neurology Emeritus
Tufts University School of Medicine
Boston, Massachusetts

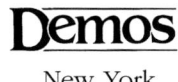
New York

Demos Medical Publishing, LLC.
386 Park Avenue South
New York, NY 10016, USA
Visit our website at www.demosmedpub.com

First edition 2005

Library of Congress Cataloging-in-Publication Data

Dystonia / [edited by] Joseph Jankovic.
        p. ; cm.
    Includes bibliographical references and index.
    ISBN-10: 1-888799-87-0; ISBN-13: 978-1-888799-87-3 (pbk. : alk. paper)
    1. Dystonia.
    [DNLM: 1. Dystonia. 2. Dystonic Disorders.] I. Jankovic, Joseph.
    RC935.D8D97 2005
    616.7'4—dc22

                                        2004031069

06 07 08 09 10   9 8 7 6 5 4 3 2

Preface

Dystonia is a neurologic disorder characterized by involuntary, sustained, patterned, and often repetitive muscle contractions of opposing muscles that cause twisting movements, abnormal postures, or both (1). One of the earliest descriptions of dystonia was provided in 1888 by Gowers, who used the term "tetanoid chorea" to describe the movement disorder in two siblings who were later diagnosed to have Wilson's disease. The term "dystonia musculorum deformans," coined by Oppenheim in 1911, was criticized for several reasons: fluctuating muscle tone was not necessarily characteristic of the disorder; the term "musculorum" incorrectly implied that the involuntary movement was due to a muscle disorder; and not all patients became deformed. More recently, the term "torsion dystonia" has been used in the literature, but since torsion is part of the definition of dystonia, this term seems redundant. Hence, the simple term "dystonia" is currently preferred and used to describe the phenomenology of this movement disorder. When used to describe a disease, it should be prefaced as either primary (without any associated neurologic deficit; it may be idiopathic or genetic) or secondary (caused by a variety of etiologies such as brain insult, certain drugs, and a variety of heredodegenerative disorders).

The primary objective of this seminar is to provide a practical review of dystonia that emphasizes cost-effective evaluation and treatment. This should be of particular value to physicians in developing countries who have limited diagnostic and therapeutic resources. Maintaining this focus is challenging in view of the increasing dependence on the latest imaging, genetic, and other technologies to evaluate patients with neurologic disorders. Furthermore, there is growing emphasis on evidence-based medicine to select only treatments that have proved efficacy and safety. However, these treatments may not be readily accessible in developing countries. For example, until recently pallidotomy, rather than medication, was the preferred treatment for Parkinson's disease in some countries, as the cost of surgery was less than long-term treatment with levodopa or dopamine agonists. A more relevant issue with respect to dystonia is the use of botulinum toxin, considered the treatment of choice for many focal or segmental dystonias (2). While relatively costly, this treatment has such important beneficial impact on the function, productivity, and quality of life of the affected individual, as demonstrated by many well-designed studies, that it may be cost-effective even in the setting of limited resources.

The contributors to this seminar have addressed these issues and balanced the advantages of the latest technologies and treatments against the practicality of the "real-world" situation facing health care providers in developing countries as they evaluate patients with dystonia and related movement disorders. I believe that the result is a collection of scholarly and, at the same time, practical reviews.

I am grateful to the authors for sharing their expertise and for providing excellent material. I also would like to thank Ted Munsat, MD for inviting me to chair this seminar and for having the confidence that the authors I selected would meet the challenge. Finally, I would like to express my appreciation to Dr. Diana M. Schneider for her constant encouragement and guidance.

Joseph Jankovic, MD

1. Jankovic J, Fahn S. Dystonic disorders. In: Jankovic J, Tolosa E, (eds.) *Parkinson's Disease and Movement Disorders*. 4th ed. Philadelphia, PA: Lippincott Williams & Wilkins. 2002:331–357.
2. Jankovic J. Botulinum toxin in clinical practice. *J Neurol Neurosurg Psychiatry*. 2004;75:951-957.

Editor's Preface

The mission of the World Federation of Neurology (WFN, wfneurology.org) is to develop international programs for the improvement of neurologic health, with an emphasis on developing countries. A major strategic aim is to develop and promote affordable and effective continuing neurologic education for neurologists and related health care providers. With this continuing education series, the WFN launches a new effort in this direction. The *WFN Seminars in Neurology* uses an instructional format that has proven to be successful in controlled trials of educational techniques. Modeled after the American Academy of Neurology's highly successful *Continuum*, we use proven pedagogical techniques to enhance the effectiveness of the course. These include case-oriented information, key points, multiple choice questions, annotated references, and abundant use of graphic material.

In addition, the course content has a special goal and direction. We live in an economic environment in which even the wealthiest nations have to restrict health care in one form or another. Especially hard pressed are countries where, of necessity, neurologic care is often reduced to the barest essentials or less. There is general agreement that much of this problem is a result of increasing technology. With this in mind, we have asked the faculty to present the instructional material and patient care guidelines with minimal use of expensive technology. Technology of unproven usefulness has not been recommended. However, at the same time, advice on patient care is given without compromising a goal of achieving the very best available care for the patient with neurologic disease. On occasion, details of certain investigative techniques are pulled out of the main text and presented separately for those interested. This approach should be of particular benefit to health care systems that are attempting to provide the best in neurologic care but with limited resources.

These courses are provided to participants by a distribution process unusual for continuing education material. The WFN membership consists of 86 individual national neurologic societies. Societies that have expressed an interest in the program and agree to meet certain specific reporting requirements are provided a limited number of courses without charge. Funding for the program is provided by unrestricted educational grants. Preference is given to neurologic societies with limited resources. Each society receiving material agrees to convene a discussion group of participants at a convenient location within a few months of receiving the material. This discussion group becomes an important component of the learning experience and has proved to be highly successful.

Our third course addresses the important area of management of the dystonias. The Chair of this course, Professor Joseph Jankovic, a recognized international authority, has selected an outstanding faculty of experts. We very much welcome your comments and advice for future courses.

Theodore L. Munsat, M.D.
Professor of Neurology Emeritus
Tufts University School of Medicine
Boston, Massachusetts

Acknowledgment

The World Federation of Neurology and faculty of this course on Dystonia gratefully acknowledge the assistance provided for its development by Allergan, and especially the assistance of Dr. G.K. Kannan.

Contents

CHAPTER 1

DIAGNOSIS, CLASSIFICATION, AND PATHOPHYSIOLOGY OF DYSTONIA

Cynthia A. Comella, MD

CASE 1

A 10-year-old boy presented with a history of progressive abnormal movements beginning 2 years previously. The first symptom observed by his parents was a limp, and inversion of the right foot that occurred when the child ran. The posture disappeared when the child walked or stood still. The movements were continuous during the day but ceased during sleep.

This patient was active in sports, and a member of the soccer and track teams. Initially, it was suspected that his symptoms were the result of a strain injury. However, splinting and rest did not improve his condition. The symptoms progressed, and the foot posturing began to occur when walking. Over the next year, posturing was noted in the entire leg and torso, with bending of the trunk to the right. During this time, his parents were having financial difficulties that caused an unstable home situation. The child's symptoms were attributed to a reaction to his stressful home environment, and he was referred to a psychiatrist for evaluation and treatment of a psychogenic disorder. Despite intensive psychotherapy, involvement of the other foot and leg occurred, resulting in an inability to walk, and the patient became wheelchair bound. Spasms affected his limbs, trunk, and neck. The child was referred to a neurologist. At the time of his examination, the boy demonstrated severe spasms with abnormal posturing of his limbs and spasms in which his trunk would arch and his head would be thrown backward. The remainder of his neurologic and physical examination was normal. His deep tendon reflexes were normal. Cognitive functioning and psychologic testing were also normal. There was no family history of any neurologic problem.

Dystonia is defined as a clinical syndrome with involuntary sustained muscle contractions that usually produce twisting and repetitive movements or abnormal postures. Symptoms particular to this syndrome help distinguish it from other movement disorders. For example, there may be overlying spasms that can appear tremorlike; in this case, the directional quality of the movement distinguishes dystonia from the tremor disorders. The movements of dystonia also tend to be slower than the rapid muscle jerks present in tic disorders. In addition, the occurrence in the foot as the initial presentation is unusual for a tic disorder, which frequently presents with eye blinks or facial jerks. Finally, dystonia characteristically exhibits a patterned movement with consistent posturing, unlike chorea, which produces rapid, unpredictable movement.

Dystonia is a clinical syndrome marked by sustained abnormal postures. It may be misdiagnosed as a psychogenic disorder by a clinician unfamiliar with its clinical features.

The diagnosis of dystonia is based entirely on the clinical examination. Currently, there is no supporting laboratory or imaging tests to confirm the diagnosis. Dystonia is traditionally classified by 1 of 3 means: distribution (body areas involved), age of onset, and etiology (Tables 1.1–1.3).

DIAGNOSIS OF DYSTONIA

The onset of dystonia in this young patient would initially have been classified as a focal dystonia with isolated involvement of the right foot. At onset, the dystonia was action dependent, with foot inversion occurring only when the child ran; it later progressed to presence at rest. This dystonia spread to become generalized dystonia with involvement of both legs, the torso, and the neck. This type of spread is common in childhood-onset dystonia.

Childhood-onset dystonia often begins in the leg and generalizes to other body regions; adult-onset dystonia usually begins in the neck or face and rarely generalizes to other body regions.

The dystonia in this patient would have been further classified as a primary dystonia because there were no additional neurologic or cognitive deficits to

TABLE 1.1   **Classification of Dystonia by Distribution**

Classification	Areas of involvement	Examples
Focal	A single body area	Eye closure (blepharospasm), neck muscles (cervical dystonia), writer's cramp (Limb dystonia), vocal cords (spasmodic dysphonia
Segmental	Two contiguous body regions	Blepharospasm and lower face or jaw (Meige syndrome)
		Cervical dystonia and writer's cramp
Generalized	One leg, trunk, and one other body region	
OR		
Both legs and trunk		Childhood onset with spread
Multifocal	Two noncontiguous body regions	Blepharospasm and foot dystonia
Hemidystonia	Body regions on one side	Arm and leg on one side of the body

TABLE 1.2   **Classification of Dystonia by Age of Onset**

Classification	Age
Childhood onset	Onset of symptoms at age <21
Adult Onset	Onset of symptoms at age >21

suggest a secondary dystonia. In the absence of these or other medical problems, no additional laboratory testing is necessary. Although DYT1 testing is commercially available, at this time, it does not alter treatment approaches and may be delayed until therapeutic modalities are specifically aimed at the DYT1 gene.

Primary dystonia is dystonia that occurs without an identifiable etiology. Patients with primary dystonia infrequently require extensive laboratory or neuroimaging studies.

If additional findings were present—such as spasticity, delayed developmental milestones, loss of milestones, cognitive impairment, or features of parkinsonism—the dystonia would then be considered a secondary dystonia and additional assessments for an underlying neurologic or metabolic disease might be indicated. These would include brain imaging, laboratory testing, and appropriate metabolic testing for pediatric disorders. A history of diurnal variation of the dystonia, with symptoms worsening over the course of the day and improvement following sleep, would suggest dopa-responsive dystonia (DRD), a disorder that is important to recognize because small doses of levodopa may provide dramatic sustained improvement. These children may have signs of parkinsonism and spasticity and be misdiagnosed as having cerebral palsy. Because levodopa may reverse most symptoms over a prolonged period of treatment, children with generalized dystonia should be given a trial of levodopa up to 600 mg per day in divided doses.

This patient was initially diagnosed as having a psychogenic dystonia. The occurrence of dystonia with particular actions, such as running, and the reduction of dystonic symptoms during sleep, may lead to a misdiagnosis of psychogenic movement disorder and subsequent attempts to identify psychologic factors that underlie symptoms. Psychotherapy is ineffective in reducing dystonia symptoms. The hallmarks of psychogenic dystonia include bizarre, inconsistent movements that are often distractible. An example of a psychogenic movement disorder would be a posturing of the fingers that varies in its appearance and disappears when complex finger tapping is performed by the other hand.

The diagnosis of drug-induced dystonia requires a history of exposure to particular medications that can cause dystonic reactions. Particularly in children, dystonic reactions may result from the use of certain antiemet-

TABLE 1.3	Classification by Etiology

Primary Dystonia

- Dystonia is the only sign without associated neurological findings.
- Evaluation does not reveal any other cause for dystonia.

Genetic

- DYT1: Onset typically in childhood with spread to become generalized dystonia. Gene isolated. Clinical testing available.
- DYT2, 4, 7, 11, 13: No clinical testing available.

Sporadic

- No family history.
- Most adult-onset dystonia. Some may have genetic basis.

Secondary Dystonia

Associated with hereditary neurologic syndromes.

1. Dystonia Plus

Dopa-responsive dystonia

- GCHI mutations (DRD or DYT5)
- Tyrosine hydroxylase mutations
- Other biopterin deficient states
- Dopamine agonist responsive dystonia due to decarboxylase deficiency
- Myoclonus—Dystonia

2. Other inherited (degenerative) disorders

- Autosomal-dominant
- Rapid-onset dystonia-parkinsonism
- Huntington's disease
- Machado-Joseph's disease/SCA3 disease
- Other SCA subtypes
- DRPLA
- Familial basal ganglia calcifications
- Autosomal-recessive
- Wilson's
- Gangliosidoses
- Metachromatic leukodystrophy
- Homocystinuria
- Hartnup disease
- Glutaric acidemia
- Methylmalonic aciduria
- Hallervorden-Spatz disease
- Dystonic lipidosis
- Ceroid-lipofuscinosis
- Ataxia-telangiectasia
- Neuroacanthocytosis
- Intraneuronal inclusion disease
- Juvenile Parkinsonism (Parkin)
- X-linked recessive
- Lubag (X-linked dystonia-parkinsonism or DYT3)
- Lesch-Nyhan syndrome
- Deafness/Dystonia
- Mitochondrial
- MERRF/MELAS
- Leber's disease

3. Due to acquired/exogenous causes

- Perinatal cerebral injury
- Encephalitis, infectious, and postinfectious
- Head trauma
- Pontine myelinolysis
- Primary antiphospholipid syndrome
- Stroke
- Tumor
- Multiple sclerosis
- Cervical cord injury or lesion
- Peripheral injury
- Drugs
- Toxins
- Psychogenic

4. Dystonia due to degenerative parkinsonian disorders

- Parkinson Disease
- Multiple system atrophy
- Progressive supranuclear palsy
- Cortico basal ganglionic degeneration

ics, such as perchlorpromazine or metoclopramide, or antipsychotics, such as haloperidol or pimozide. These usually present with forced eye deviations and involuntary trunk and neck extensions (oculogyric crisis), and are infrequently confused with primary dystonia. Acute drug-induced dystonic reactions are transient, resolving with drug discontinuation, and are acutely responsive to anticholinergic administration. However, the chronic administration of the same class of dopamine receptor antagonist drugs may cause tardive dystonia, which may be either focal or generalized and often presents as trunk and neck extension, sometimes associated with stereotypic mouth movements. Tardive dystonia is chronic and persists with discontinuation of the offending drug. The history of a temporal relationship of the onset of dystonia following sustained use of these drugs suggests this diagnosis.

The list of the genetic forms of dystonia has expanded greatly over the past decade. The most frequent genetic form of dystonia with childhood onset and secondary generalization is DYT1 dystonia. In youth-onset primary dystonia, especially in Ashkenazi Jews, this is the most common genetic form of dystonia. Although inherited in an autosomal-dominant fashion, the penetrance of the gene is reduced, and only 30%–40% of those carrying the gene will have symptoms of dystonia. This means that, despite the absence of a family history of dystonia in this patient, it is likely that the patient will have a genetic form of dystonia, and may have the DYT1 gene. This gene is located on chromosome 9, in the 9q32-34 region. It is a GAG deletion that gives rise to a deletion in a glutamic acid residue in a protein called torsin A. The function of torsin A has not been elucidated, but it is widely distributed in the brain. Most patients with dystonia due to DYT1 have symptom onset before the age of 26 years, with 1 or more limbs affected. Testing for DYT1 is recommended for patients with dystonia onset before the age of 26 years, and in those with onset over the age of 26, but with a relative who has early-onset dystonia. This patient would fall within the guidelines for obtaining DYT1 testing, if affordable. Genetic counseling for the patient and family would be also recommended if available.

In summary, this patient had the typical history and physical findings of youth-onset primary dystonia. In the absence of any other associated neurologic abnormalities and no other putative cause for dystonia, a trial of levodopa would be recommended to rule out the possibility of dopa-responsive dystonia.

No other testing is essential. Obtaining a DYT1 gene test would clarify whether the patient had this one form of inherited dystonia, but would not be useful in diagnosing the dystonic syndrome.

A trial of levodopa is recommended in childhood-onset dystonia, or in adults with generalized dystonia, especially if accompanied by additional neurologic abnormalities such as parkinsonism or spasticity.

CASE 2

A 42-year-old woman presented with right-sided neck pain that started 3 years previously. She initially attributed the pain to a stiff neck or arthritis. However, the pain increased in intensity and she noticed that her head tended to move to the right. She felt that movement to the left was restricted. Over the following year, the movement to the right became more pronounced, and was observed by her coworkers. When attempting to hold her head in a forward position, she would have a side-to-side tremor. If she touched her chin, or held her head in her hand, her movements would abate. She developed an ulnar neuropathy from resting her head on her left hand with her elbow on the table. Over the past year, she also reported difficulties with her handwriting. Although not occurring during any other activity with her right hand, when trying to write, she noticed that her second and third fingers would bend forward and that her hand would tend to supinate. There was no family history of similar problems, although a maternal aunt had developed tremor in both hands when she was 60 years old. Neurologic examination of this patient was remarkable for head posturing to the right with an elevation of the right shoulder, and ulnar neuropathy on the left. There was neither tremor nor bradykinesia in the limbs. When writing, flexion of the index and third finger occurred, with flexion at the wrist and internal rotation of the arm.

In contrast to the first patient, this patient developed symptoms in mid-adulthood. Her first symptom was pain localized to an area of her neck. Involuntary, sustained turning of her head, tremor, and writing difficulties followed. This patient had a history typical for cervical dystonia (CD) with subsequent development of writer's cramp.

CD is a focal dystonia with involvement of the neck muscles. Previously known as spasmodic torticollis, it is a common form of adult-onset dystonia with occurrence of symptoms in the fifth decade. CD is 1.5 to 3 times more common in women than in men. It usually remains localized to the neck area, though it may spread to a contiguous body area as it did in this patient, and become part of a segmental dystonia. As is true with all adult-onset focal dystonias, it is rare for this dystonia to become generalized.

Head postures associated with CD vary. There may be a turning of the head (torticollis) to one side, a lateral flexion of the neck (laterocollis), a forward flexion of the head (anterocollis), or a posterior extension of the head (retrocollis). There may also be a shifting of the head on the shoulders in a sagittal plane. In many patients, the movement is not a single movement, but rather a combination of the above. In addition, there may be overlying muscle spasms, as were observed in this patient, causing quick, repetitive jerking movements that may be mistaken for essential tremor. Although there may be an association of essential tremor with dystonia, in this patient the directional preponderance of the movement to the right, along with the positional quality of the tremor—only occurring when turning to the left—suggest this to be a dystonic tremor.

Cervical pain occurs in as many as 60% of patients with CD, and may be the most disabling feature of this disease. Although pain may derive directly from dystonia, other causes include cervical arthritis and radiculopathy. Some patients report pain in the suboccipital region radiating unilaterally into the scalp. This suggests an occipital neuralgia that may arise due to compression of the greater occipital nerve as it emerges from the base of the skull to provide sensory innervation for the top of the head.

Among the most interesting features of dystonia is the presence of the geste antagoniste, or "sensory trick," that occurs in many patients with focal dystonia. This is a gesture or touch that can transiently alleviate the symptoms of dystonia. In CD, patients will find that a touch to the cheek or the back of the head allows them to bring their head forward. Electromyogram shows reduction in dystonic muscle activity when performing a sensory trick. The presence of these tricks sometimes leads inaccurately to a misdiagnosis of a psychogenic movement disorder. However, the presence of them is one of the hallmarks of dystonia.

CD is the most common dystonia seen in referral centers, but is relatively rare, with an estimated prevalence of approximately 90 to 120 per 1 million persons. Other common types of focal dystonia with onset in adulthood include blepharospasm, spasmodic dysphonia, and writer's cramp. If this patient had initially developed a focal dystonia in the leg, it would have strongly suggested that the dystonia was secondary. Adult-onset focal foot dystonia may be the first symptom of young-onset Parkinson's disease or symptomatic of a structural lesion in the spinal cord or brain. CD with predominant anterocollis can be seen in patients with multiple system atrophy, but is rarely a presenting feature of the disorder.

Primary CD is rare in infancy and childhood, usually occurring secondary to other disorders. In infancy,

the most common cause of torticollis is congenital muscular torticollis, with shortening of a sternocleidomastoid muscle, causing a head tilt. Other causes of torticollis developing in infancy include intrauterine crowding, malformations of the cervical spine, and Arnold–Chiari malformations. In childhood, torticollis is usually caused by either cervical abnormalities or rotational atlantoaxial subluxation. Nasopharyngeal infections and posterior fossa and cervical cord lesions are other local causes of torticollis. Abnormal posturing of the head may occur to compensate for visual disturbances such as diplopia or congenital nystagmus. Sandifer's syndrome arising from gastroesophageal reflux and esophagitis should also be considered. Although onset of torticollis in adulthood is almost always primary, CD may arise as a tardive syndrome following exposure to dopamine receptor antagonists. Torticollis occurring at any age with sudden onset, severe pain, restricted range of movement, and no improvement during sleep is likely to have originated from an underlying structural lesion.

The pathophysiology of focal dystonia is not known. Electrophysiologic studies suggest loss of central inhibitory mechanisms. Imaging studies suggest abnormalities in the lenticular nucleus and dorsal striatum. Modulation of CD symptoms by gesture or touch (geste antagoniste) suggests involvement of sensory input.

Although most cases of CD appear to be sporadic, clinical investigations have suggested that an autosomal-dominant genetic mutation with reduced penetrance is responsible for this disease in many patients. The DYT1 gene has been excluded as a cause of familial CD. Both DYT6 (chromosome 8) and DYT7 (chromosome 18p) have been identified as possible loci in large families with CD. This disease is likely to be genetically heterogeneous, as both DYT6 and DYT7 have been ruled out in several large families.

This patient also had dystonia of her hand manifested as writer's cramp. Task-specific dystonia is dystonia that occurs only during the performance of specific tasks, such as writing. The task that causes the dystonia may vary in different patients. A piano player may have dystonia only while trying to play certain sequences of keys, a typist may have dystonia while typing but not with writing, or a woodwind player may develop dystonia of the mouth or jaw only while playing his or her instrument (embouchure dystonia). Task-specific dystonias are not understood, although they have been hypothesized to arise from overuse of the limb in question.

In summary, this patient demonstrated the typical features of adult-onset CD with subsequent spread to the hand as segmental dystonia. Unless unusual features are present, additional workup is rarely neces-

---

Treatment of dystonia is symptom oriented, and includes pharmacologic agents, chemodenervation with botulinum toxin, and surgical approaches.

---

sary. Treatment of focal dystonia has largely been through chemodenervation of the overactive dystonic muscles, using botulinum toxin. This procedure, however, is expensive and needs to be repeated at approximately 3- to 4-month intervals. If botulinum toxin treatment is not available, pharmacologic agents—specifically, anticholinergic drugs, baclofen, clonazepam, and tetrabenazine—may be tried, although the success of these treatments is often limited by the occurrence of adverse effects. Bilateral deep-brain stimulation surgery has been observed recently to be effective for symptoms of dystonia. Some experts have suggested that bilateral pallidotomy may be just as effective, although with ablative surgery, possible complications including dysarthria, cognitive change, and spasticity are not reversible.

CASE 3

A 56-year-old woman with a history of hypertension presented with dystonic posturing of her right arm and leg. The symptoms began suddenly approximately 1 month earlier and had been stable since onset. She had difficulty using her right hand, and found that she was unable to write. She also had problems with right foot inversion that caused pain and swelling in the ankle joint. She had had no previous problems with involuntary movements. Her family history was negative for dystonia.

Her neurologic examination showed inversion of the right foot with extension of the great toe. There was an internal rotation of the leg at the right hip. Her right arm was flexed at the elbow and wrist, with the fingers of the hand flexed at the metacarpophalangeal and proximal interphalangeal joints. There was a mild hyperreflexia of the right side. Sensory examination was normal. She was able to walk only with assistance. The diagnosis was hemidystonia. A magnetic resonance imaging scan showed an infarct in the left putamen.

In contrast to primary dystonia, symptomatic dystonia is often associated with lesions involving the basal ganglia. In particular, pathologic processes of the putamen are most likely to give rise to hemidystonia in the contralateral body. Lesions in other areas have also been associated with dystonia, including those located in the thalamus, cortex, cerebellum, brainstem, and spinal cord. Secondary blepharospasm has been observed following an infarct of the upper brainstem. The most common pathologic lesion observed is infarction, although tumors and vascular malformations may also be associated with this dystonia.

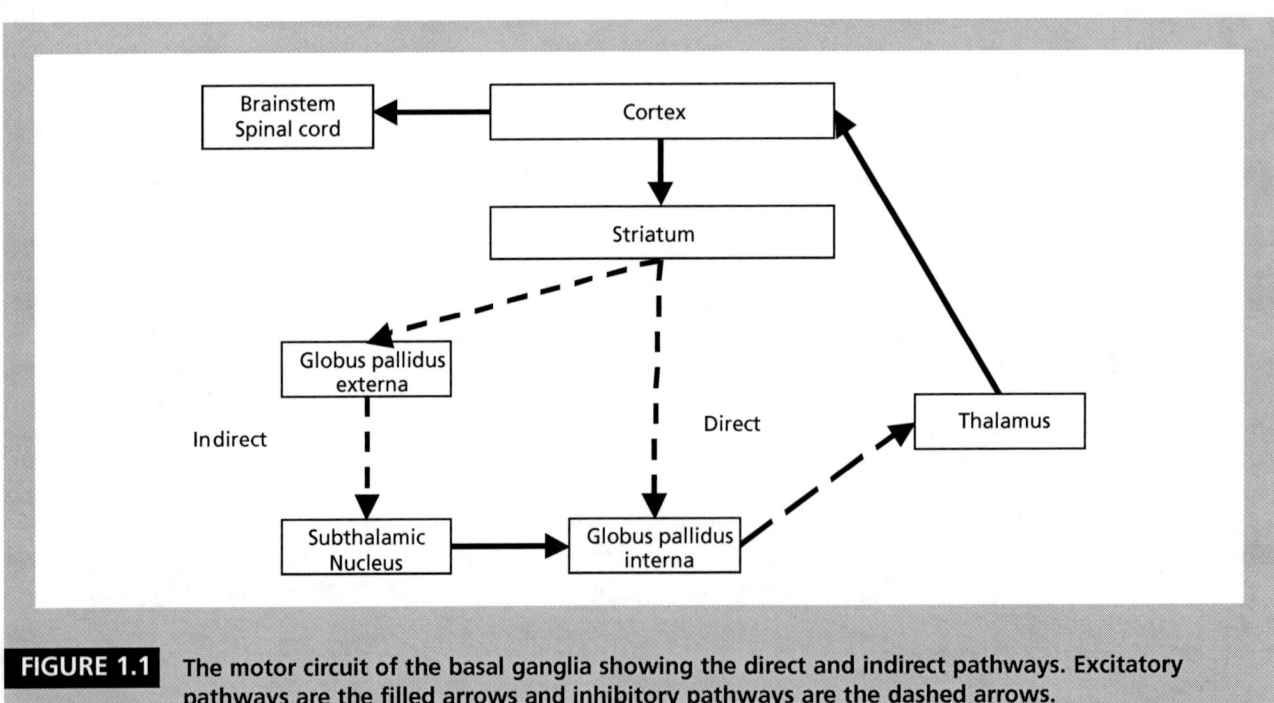

FIGURE 1.1 The motor circuit of the basal ganglia showing the direct and indirect pathways. Excitatory pathways are the filled arrows and inhibitory pathways are the dashed arrows.

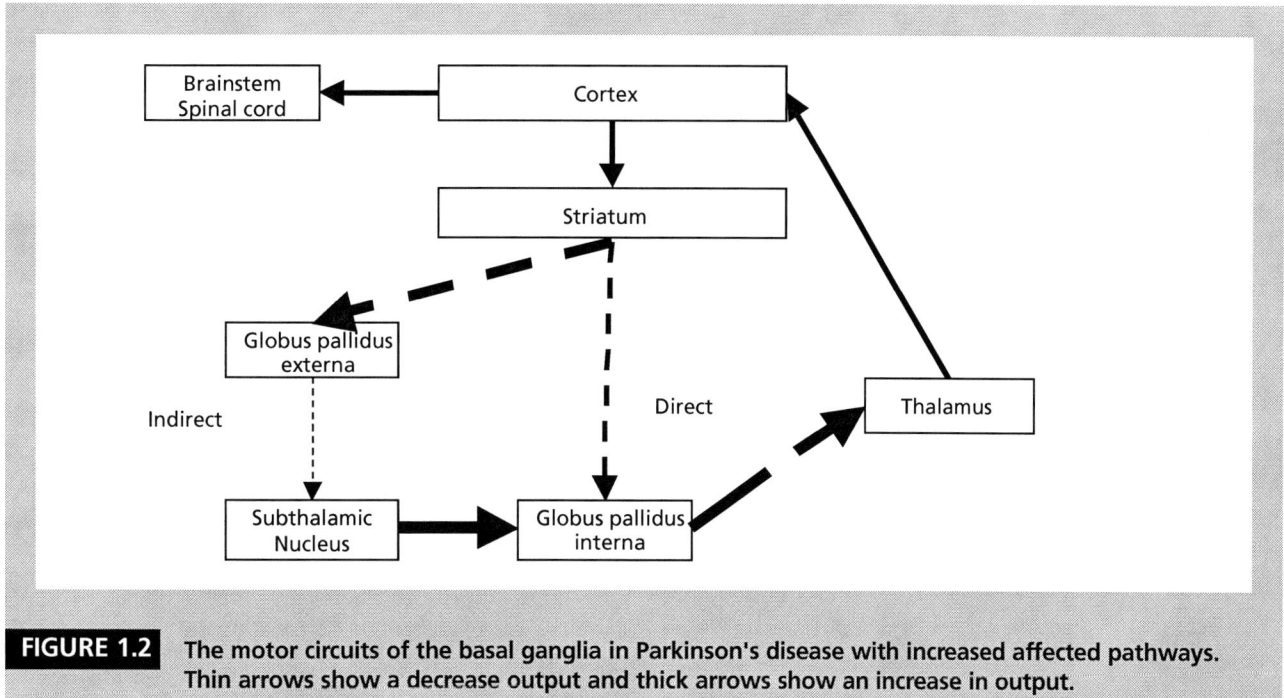

FIGURE 1.2 The motor circuits of the basal ganglia in Parkinson's disease with increased affected pathways. Thin arrows show a decrease output and thick arrows show an increase in output.

The description of hemidystonia secondary to basal ganglia lesions provides an invaluable clue as to the underlying anatomy of the dystonia. The basal ganglia have dense fiber connections to the thalamus and the cerebral cortex. The motor loops of the basal ganglia include direct and indirect pathways (Figure 1.1). The direct pathway flows from the striatum directly to the globus pallidus internus (GPi) and inhibits it. The indirect pathway flows from the striatum to the globus pallidus externa to the subthalamic nucleus and has an excitatory effect on the GPi. The primary outflow from the basal ganglia to the thalamus is an inhibitory path-

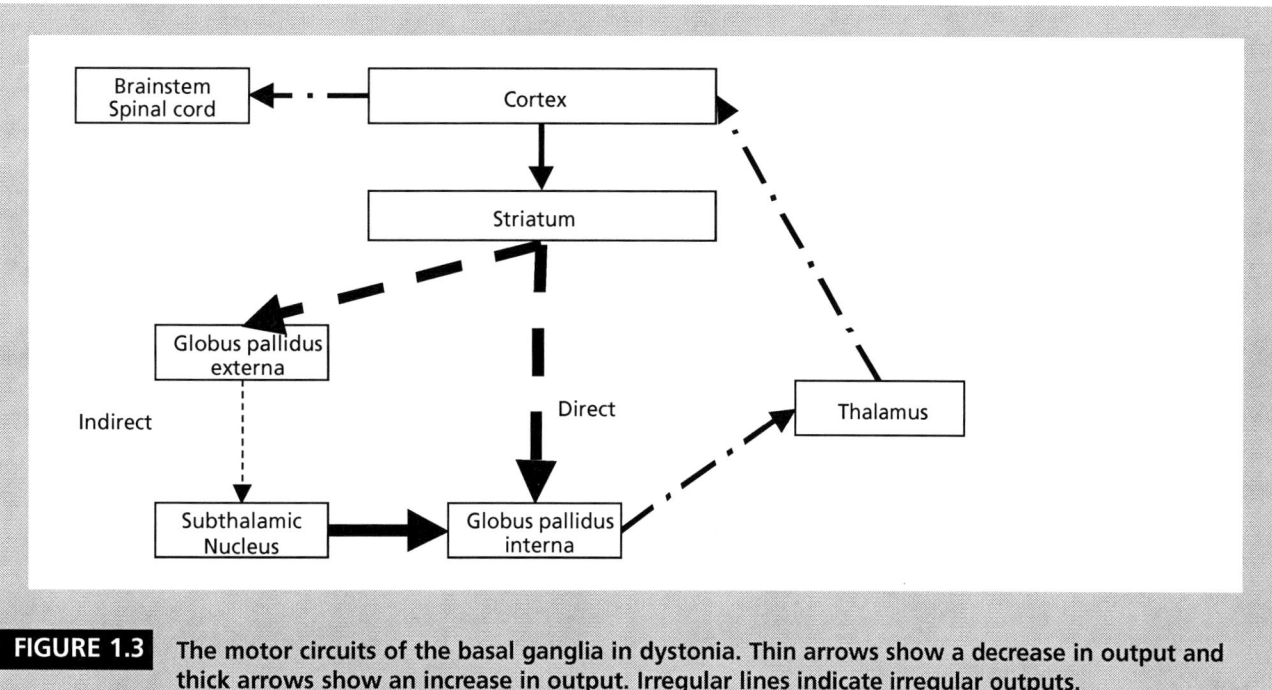

FIGURE 1.3 The motor circuits of the basal ganglia in dystonia. Thin arrows show a decrease in output and thick arrows show an increase in output. Irregular lines indicate irregular outputs.

way originating from the GPi. Parkinson disease is mediated primarily through an increase in the excitatory effect of the indirect pathway, causing an increase in GPi inhibition of the thalamus. In contrast, dystonia is hypothesized to involve both direct and indirect pathways, causing abnormalities in discharge rates and pattern of firing of the GPi neurons.

To summarize, this patient had a symptomatic hemidystonia with an infarction in the contralateral basal ganglia. It was through investigations of similar patients that researchers had the first glimmer of understanding of the underlying pathophysiology and anatomy of dystonia.

In progressive dystonia associated with cognitive or psychiatric features, testing for Wilson's disease is necessary.

In patients with other forms of secondary dystonia, a careful history and physical and neurologic examination are essential to investigate for the underlying cause. An important secondary dystonia to consider is Wilson's disease. To assess for this disease, a slit lamp examination for Kayser–Fleischer rings, a serum ceruloplasmin, and a 24-hour urine test for copper are recommended. A patient with Wilson's disease may be treated successfully by chelation therapy.

ADDITIONAL READING

Bressman S. Dystonia update. *Clin Neuropharmacol* 2000;23:239–251.

Bressman SB, Sabatti C, Raymond D, de Leon D, Klein C, Kramer PL, et al. The DYT1 phenotype and guidelines for diagnostic testing. *Neurology* 2000;54:1746–1752.

Chan J, Brin MF, Fahn S. Idiopathic cervical dystonia: clinical characteristics. *Mov Disord* 1991;6:119–126.

Claypool DW. Epidemiology and outcome of cervical dystonia (spasmodic torticollis) in Rochester, Minnesota. *Mov Disord* 1995;10:608–614.

Eidelberg D, Moeller JR, Antonini A, Dhawan V, Spetsieris P, de Leon D, et al. Functional brain networks in DYT1 dystonia. *Ann Neurol* 1998;44:303–312.

Epidemiologic Study of Dystonia in Europe (ESDE) Collaborative Group. Sex-related influences on the frequency and age of onset of primary dystonia. *Neurology* 1999;53:1871–1873.

Fahn S, Bressman SB, Marsden CD. Classification of dystonia. *Adv Neurol* 1998;78:1–10.

Fahn S, Marsden CD, Calne DB. Classification and investigation of dystonia. In: Marsden CD, Fahn S, (eds.) *Movement Disorders 2*. London: Butterworth and Co; 1987:332–358.

Greene P, Kang UJ, Fahn S. Spread of symptoms in idiopathic dystonia. *Mov Disord* 1995;10:143–152.

Jankovic J, Fahn S. Dystonic disorders. In: Jankovic J, Tolosa E, (eds.) *Parkinson's Disease and Movement Disorders*. 2nd ed. Baltimore: Williams & Wilkins; 1993:337–374.

Kaji R. Basal ganglia as a sensory gating device for motor control. *J Med Invest* 2001;48:142–146.

Kostic VS, Stojanovic-Svetel M, Kacar A. Symptomatic dystonias associated with brain structural lesions: report of 16 cases. *Can J Neurol Sci* 1996;23:53–56.

Kramer LP, de Leon D, Ozelius L, Risch NJ, Bressman SB, Brin MF, et al. Dystonia gene in Ashkenazi Jewish population is located in chromosome 9q32-34. *Ann Neurol* 1990;27:114–120.

Lowenstein DH, Aminoff MJ. The clinical course of spasmodic torticollis. *Neurology* 1988;38:530–532.

Marsden CD, Obeso JA, Zarranz JJ, Lang AE. The anatomical basis of symptomatic hemidystonia. *Brain* 1985;108:463–483.

Muller J, Wissel J, Masuhr F, Ebersbach G, Wenning GK, Poewe W. Clinical characteristics of the geste antagoniste in cervical dystonia. *J Neurol* 2001;248:478–482.

Nutt JG, Muenter MD, Aronson A, Kurland LT, Melton LJ. Epidemiology of focal and generalized dystonia in Rochester, Minnesota. *Movement Dis* 1988;3:188–194.

Nygaard TG, Trugman JM, de Yebenes JG, Fahn S. Dopa-responsive dystonia: the spectrum of clinical manifestations in a large North American family. *Neurology* 1990;40:66–69.

Ozelius L, Kramer PL, Moskowitz CB, Kwiatkowski DJ, Brin MF, Bressman SB, et al. Human gene for torsion dystonia located on chromosome 9q32-34. *Neuron* 1989;2:1427–1434.

Suchowersky O, Calne DB. Non-dystonic causes of torticollis. *Adv Neurol* 1988;50:501–508.

Vitek JL. Pathophysiology of dystonia: a neuronal model. *Mov Disord* 2002;17(suppl 3):S49–S62.

Vitek JL, Chockkan V, Zhang JY, Kaneoke Y, Evatt M, DeLong MR, et al. Neuronal activity in the basal ganglia in patients with generalized dystonia and hemiballism. *Ann Neurol* 1999;46:22–35.

CHAPTER 2

THE GENETICS OF DYSTONIA

M. Tagliati, MD, M. Pourfar, MD, and Susan B. Bressman, MD

INTRODUCTION

Dystonia comprises a heterogeneous group of disorders characterized by sustained and involuntary muscle contractions generally resulting in an abnormal twisting posture. These disorders have been divided into primary (or idiopathic) and secondary (or symptomatic) subsets. Since Ozelius and colleagues first described a mutation in the DYT1 gene in 1989, the genetic underpinnings of many of the dystonias have become evident. There are currently more than a dozen genetic loci associated with the clinical expression of dystonia, and the number of other genes associated with dystonic disorders continues to grow steadily. Despite this growing body of information, the majority of genes that cause primary dystonias have yet to be identified. This overview will focus on the present delineation of genetically associated primary dystonias along with some of the "dystonia-plus" syndromes in which other features may coexist with the dystonia. Table 2.1 outlines the major genetic loci associated with dystonia. The discussion here will focus mainly on the more common and better-described types, namely DYT1, DYT6, DYT7, and DYT13 in the "pure" dystonia group; DYT5, DYT11, and DYT12 in the "dystonia-plus" group; and PKD and PKND in the paroxysmal dystonia group. Figure 2.1 illustrates the chromosomal locations of the most common genetic defects associated with dystonia. Several extensive reviews in the "Additional Reading" section provide more coverage of the broad range of genetic dystonia.

TABLE 2.1 **Classification of Genetic Loci Associated with Dystonia**

Gene Locus	Location	Inheritance	Phenotype	Gene Product
DYT1	9q34	AD	Early limb–onset PTD	TorsinA
DYT2	Not mapped	AR	Early onset	
DYT3	Xq13.1	XR	Lubag dystonia/parkinsonism	Multiple transcript system
DYT4	Not mapped	AD	Whispering dysphonia	
DYT5	14q22.1	AD	DRD/parkinsonism	GCH1
DYT6	8p21-p22	AD	"mixed" cranial/cervical/limb onset	Not identified
DYT7	18p	AD	Adult cervical	Not identified
DYT8	2q33-25	AD	PDC/PNKD	Myofibrillogenesis regulator 1
DYT9	1p21	AD	Episodic choreoathetosis/ataxia with spasticity	Not identified
DYT10	16	AD	PKC/PKD (EKD1 and 2)	Not identified
DYT11	7q21	AD	Myoclonus dystonia	ε-sarcoglycan
DYT12	19q	AD	Rapid-onset dystonia parkinsonism	Na+/K+ ATPase α3
DYT13	1p36	AD	Cervical/cranial/brachial	Not identified
DYT14	14q13	AD	DRD	Not identified

AD=Autosomal dominant; DRD=dopa-resistant dystonia; EKD=Endokinin D; PDC=Paroxysmal dystonic choreathetosis; PKC=Paroxysmal kinesigenic choreathetosis; PKD=paroxysmal kinesigenic dystonia/dyskinesia; PNKD=paroxysmal nonkinesigenic dystonia/dyskinesia; PTD=Primary torsion dystonia; XR= X-linked recessive.

In addition to the general subdivision into primary and secondary forms, dystonia can be also classified by age of onset (early vs adult) and by the extent of muscle involvement and disability (generalized, focal, and mixed types). When viewed from a genetic perspective, it can be appreciated that the same mutation can cause varying phenotypes in different individuals both in terms of age of onset and localization. When studied on pathologic examination, primary dystonias are generally characterized by a lack of consistent neurodegenerative or neurochemical changes. They are also unified (with the notable exception of dopa-responsive dystonia [DRD]) by a lack of consistently efficacious pharmacologic treatment. However, recent experience supports pallidal deep brain stimulation (DBS) as a safe and efficacious treatment, in particular for patients with primary dystonia.

PRIMARY DYSTONIAS

Dystonic muscle contractions are the only neurologic abnormality in primary dystonias, and evaluation does not reveal an identifiable exogenous cause or other inherited or degenerative disease. Primary dystonias can be further classified (Table 2.2) according to their prevalent age of onset as:

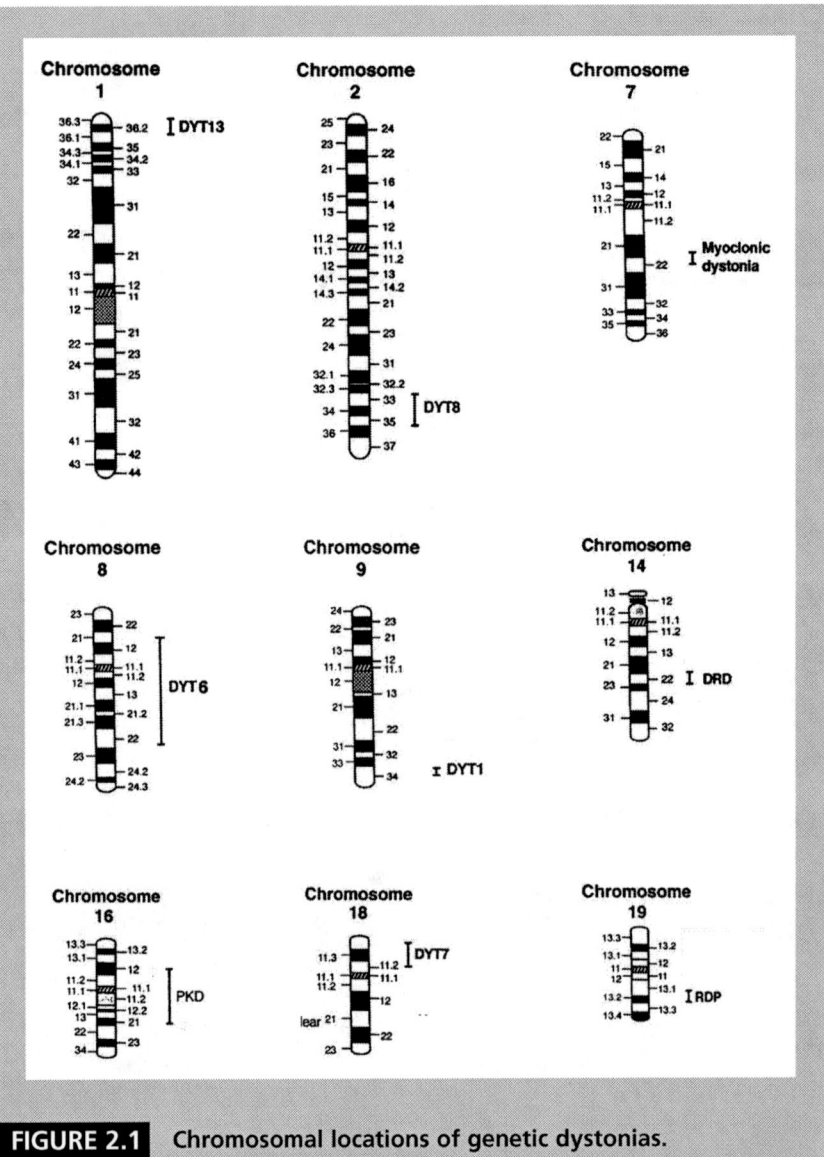

FIGURE 2.1 Chromosomal locations of genetic dystonias.

1. Childhood and adolescent onset (DYT1 and other genes to be identified), characterized by early limb onset and frequent spread to other muscles.
2. Adult onset (DYT7 and other genes to be identified), characterized by onset in cervical, cranial, or brachial muscles and limited spread.
3. Mixed phenotype (DYT6, DYT13, and other genes to be identified).

DYT1

The gene responsible for the most common of the genetically identifiable dystonias was described by Ozelius and colleagues in 1989 and named DYT1 (or TOR1A). The defect leading to dystonia is a deletion of an inframe GAG trinucleotide localized to chromosome 9q32-34. The DYT1 gene encodes torsinA, a protein expressed throughout the central nervous system that belongs to the family of AAA+ proteins (ATPases associated with a variety of activities).

These proteins often serve as chaperones and are involved in a variety of functions, including protein folding and degradation, cytoskeletal dynamics, membrane trafficking and vesicle fusion, and response to stress. The function of torsinA remains elusive and the mechanism(s) by which mutant torsinA may compromise neuronal function are unknown, but may include an altered response to stress-induced changes in protein structure. Neuronal degeneration has not been identified in the brains of patients with DYT1 dystonia. Although brainstem neuronal inclusino have recently been described.

TABLE 2.2   Etiologic Classification of Dystonia

Primary

Dystonia is the only neurologic sign. Evaluation does not reveal an identifiable exogenous cause or other inherited or degenerative disease.

Childhood and adolescent onset

- DYT1: Autosomal dominant with reduced penetrance (~30%), early limb onset with predominant family phenotype
- Other genes to be identified

Adult onset

- DYT7: Autosomal dominant, cervical onset in adult life
- Other genes to be identified

Mixed phenotype

- DYT6, DYT 13: Autosomal dominant, early and late onset with possible cranial, cervical, and sometimes limb onset and variable spread
- Other genes to be identified

Secondary

Variety of lesions, mostly involving the basal ganglia and/or dopamine synthesis.

Inherited nondegenerative (dystonia plus)

- Dopa-responsive dystonia: due to DYT5 and other genetic defects
- Myoclonus dystonia: due to DYT11 and possibly other genetic defects
- Rapid-onset dystonia parkinsonism: due to DYT12

Inherited degenerative

- Autosomal dominant, autosomal recessive, X-linked (DYT3), mitochondrial

Degenerative disorders of unknown etiology

- Parkinson disease
- Progressive supranuclear palsy
- Corticobasal ganglionic degeneration

Acquired

- Drugs (dopamine-receptor blockers), other toxins
- Head trauma
- Stroke, hypoxia
- Encephalitis, infectious and postinfectious
- Tumors
- Peripheral injuries

Other movement disorders with dystonic phenomenology

- Tics, paroxysmal dyskinesias (DYT8, DYT9, DYT10)

Psychogenic Dystonia

The same GAG deletion is responsible for dystonia in families and patients from diverse ethnic groups (Table 2.3). In the Ashkenazi population, dystonia due to DYT1 has an estimated prevalence between 1/3000 and 1/9000 with a carrier frequency of 1/1000 to 1/3000. This represents as much as a 10-fold increased prevalence as that found in the non-Ashkenazi population. The increased frequency in Ashkenazi Jews is thought to be the result of a founder mutation that was introduced into the population approximately 350 years ago, originating in the area of Lithuania or Byelorussia. The pattern of inheritance is autosomal dominant, with 30% penetrance. Thus, first-degree relatives of affected individuals have a 15% risk and second-degree relatives have about a 7%–8% risk of developing the disorder. In this population, the TOR1A GAG deletion accounts for an estimated 80%–90% of early limb–onset cases. Unlike that observed in the Ashkenazi population, the DYT1 mutation is a less common cause of early limb–onset primary dystonia in the non-Ashkenazi population, constituting about 30%–50% of the cases. There is no known founder effect and clearly other genes, yet to be identified, are important in non-Jewish populations.

Clinical expression of the DYT1 GAG deletion is generally similar across ethnic groups. While there is marked clinical variability, the disorder characteristically first affects an arm or leg beginning in mid to late childhood. Ultimately, more than 95% of patients experience involvement of the arm, while less than 15% develop cranial or cervical involvement. Patients with leg onset tend to be younger at onset and are more likely to progress to generalized dystonia compared with those with initial involvement of the arm. Progressive spread of dystonia to involve multiple muscle groups as generalized or multifocal dystonia is

TABLE 2.3   DYT1 Features in Ashkenazi and Non-Jewish Populations

	Ashkenazi	Non-Jewish
Mode of inheritance	100% AD	85% AD
Penetrance	30%	40% (in AD)
9q haplotype	Yes	No
GAG TOR1A deletion	90%	40%–65%
% new mutation	Rare	14%
Incidence	1/6000–1/2000	1/160,000
Age of onset >40 years	Uncommon	10%–15%

AD=autosomal dominant.

observed in about 65% of patients; about 25% remain focal and 10% are segmental.

CASE 1

KW had normal psychomotor development until age 7, when she initially showed turning in of her feet and posturing of the legs with prolonged walking. She subsequently developed difficulty writing and marked loss of trunk control, with difficulty maintaining erect sitting position, inability to transfer from sitting to standing position, and inability to control the left arm due to constant shoulder movements. Fixed equinovarus deformity of the left foot and varus posture of the right foot ensued over a period of 2 or 3 years. She demonstrated little response to a variety of medications, including levodopa, anticholinergics, baclofen, and benzodiazepines. Neurologic examination revealed cervical dystonia with head turning to the left, bilateral arm dystonia at rest with internal rotation, spasmodic back arching of the trunk, and dystonic flexion of the right leg at the knee and of the left foot. Brain magnetic resonance imaging (MRI) was normal. Genetic testing revealed that she was a carrier of the DYT1 mutation.

With the identification of the DYT1 gene, it is now possible to diagnose one of the most frequent causes of generalized dystonia. The DYT1 GAG deletion accounts for a significant proportion of early-onset (<26 years of age) primary dystonia. As all cases of DYT1 dystonia are due to the same GAG deletion, screening is relatively easy and commercially available. The test should be considered for all patients with primary dystonia with onset by age 26 and for individuals with later-onset dystonia who have an early-onset blood relative. DYT1 testing (when positive) will obviate other expensive diagnostic tests, including MRI, unless there are other findings on exam to suggest an independent central nervous system (CNS) or spinal cord lesion. We recommend preliminary genetic counseling when DYT1 diagnostic and carrier testing are employed.

After 6 years of disease, KW was wheelchair bound. After the failure of all available medications for dystonia, she underwent bilateral implant of pallidal DBS electrodes. Progressive and sustained improvement of dystonia was noted over the following months. The patient was able to walk and run 18 months after DBS surgery. She was practically dystonia free when stimulated. Moreover, she was able to completely discontinue her medications. We as well as other researchers have reported that in select cases of intractable primary dystonia, including DYT1-positive cases, DBS may be a safe and effective alternative over current best medical management.

DYT6

This type of primary dystonia is referred to as a mixed type because of the varying body distribution and age at onset of the dystonia within affected families. Described in 2 Mennonite families, it has been mapped to chromosome 8 (8p21-8q22). It is autosomal dominant with decreased penetrance, and appears to be the result of a founder mutation. About 1/2 of affected family members had onset of symptoms in childhood, with the rest exhibiting symptoms during the third and fourth decades. There was a wide range of body regions first affected (arm, cranial muscles, neck, and leg), and almost all had some degree of spread—or progression of dystonia—to other body regions, but again this varied widely. Most had cervical and cranial involvement, and for the majority, the greatest disability stemmed from dystonia of the neck and cranial muscles, including speech involvement.

DYT7

Leube and colleagues first described this primary focal dystonia locus in a large German family in 1996. The gene was localized to the short arm of chromosome 18. Focal in nature, it manifests primarily as cervical dystonia (familial torticollis). The age of onset varies from the second to seventh decade, with an average age of 43 years.

DYT13

This relatively indolent, typically segmental dystonia has been identified in 1 Italian family and has been mapped to the short arm of chromosome 1. It is an autosomal-dominant disorder with reduced penetrance and begins between ages 5 and 40 years. This dystonia is often limited to the cranial, neck, and/or upper limbs muscles, but can occasionally generalize.

SECONDARY DYSTONIAS

This group is comprised of disorders in which dystonia is often accompanied by other neurologic manifestations such as parkinsonism and myoclonus. They can be inherited, acquired, psychogenic, or of unknown etiology (Table 2.2). The inherited forms that are relevant for this chapter can be further classified as:

1. Inherited nondegenerative or "dystonia plus," including DRD due to DYT5 and other genetic defects; myoclonus dystonia due to DYT11 and possibly other genetic defects; and rapid-onset dystonia parkinsonism (RPD) due to DYT12.
2. Inherited degenerative, which can have an autosomal-dominant, autosomal-recessive, X-linked, or mitochondrial pattern of inheritance.

3. Paroxysmal dyskinesias (DYT8, DYT9, DYT10), which are frequently categorized separately from dystonia but which have been assigned DYT loci.

DRD (DYT5)

DRD is a form of dystonia whose hallmark feature is a remarkable response to low dosages of levodopa. The most common cause of DRD is mutation in the gene encoding guanosine triphosphate cyclohydrolase 1 (GCH1) on chromosome 14 (see Figure 2.2). DRD due to GCH1 mutations is autosomal dominant (mutations are heterozygous), and penetrance appears to be influenced by gender, being higher in females. A less common autosomal-recessive variant of DRD involves the tyrosine hydroxylase gene on chromosome 11.

Typically, DRD due to GCH1 mutations (DYT5) begins in early childhood and presents with limb or truncal dystonia, a dystonic-spastic–appearing gait, and mild parkinsonism (bradykinesia and postural instability). Onset in infancy mimicking cerebral palsy may also occur. Hyperreflexia and diurnal fluctuation of symptoms, with progressive deterioration during the day, are common. Affected individuals are all characterized by a dramatic and sustained response to levodopa, and an excellent response to cholinergic medications has also been described. The diagnosis of DRD depends on both the clinical findings and a dramatic response to low-dose levodopa therapy. Total daily dosages of as little as 50 to 200 mg of levodopa usually result in complete or near-complete reversal of symptoms and signs, which is maintained without fluctuations.

CASE 2

AS was born by normal, spontaneous, vaginal delivery, with the first four months of gestation complicated by maternal vaginal bleeding. The patient had normal cognitive development. When she began walking at the age of 9 1/2 months, her parents noticed that she had a clumsy gait, and that her toes turned inward. By age 10, she had had bilateral achilles tendon releases because of dystonic posturing of her feet. At age 11, she was diagnosed with DRD after responding well to a trial with levodopa. She continued to do well throughout puberty and was able to compete in running races. At age 13, she first experienced subtle extra movements after taking the medications. Her Sinemet (carbidopa-levodopa) dose was reduced from 350 mg/day to 200 mg/day with resolution of her abnormal movements. By age 20, she was taking only 1 Sinemet 25/100 per day. At age 25, she continued to do very well. On examination, she had minimal clumsiness when performing rapid successive movements of the left foot. She was maintained on 1 Sinemet 25/100 per day and continued to complain of left toe curling and cramping under physical exertion.

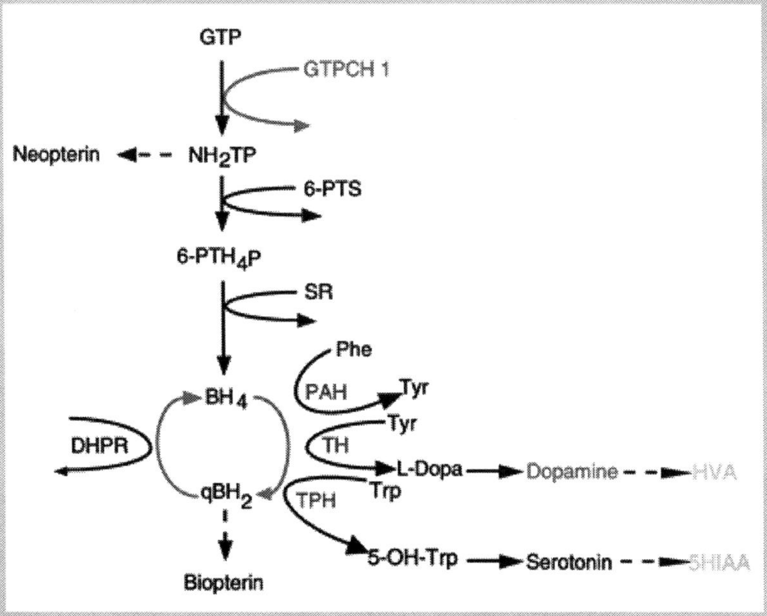

FIGURE 2.2 Diagram of GCH1 defect pathway.

Although both Parkinson's disease and DRD respond symptomatically to levodopa, the 2 differ both pathophysiologically and in their response to Sinemet. In contrast to Parkinson's disease, DRD is a nondegenerative condition and DRD patients do not usually experience clinically significant fluctuations, dyskinesias, or decreasing dosage efficacy after long-term treatment with levodopa.

Familial Myoclonus Dystonia (DYT11)

Although very rapid dystonic jerks can be part of the clinical manifestations of DYT1 and other primary dystonias, myoclonus dystonia is a distinct genetic disorder in which dystonia, usually mild and not always present, is associated with marked myoclonus. There are no other neurologic signs. Myoclonus dystonia is autosomal dominant with reduced penetrance, especially when transmitted maternally, and with variable expression, with males and females equally affected in most families. In many identified familial cases, the disease is linked to a locus on chromosome 7q21 (DYT11) and caused by mutations in the E-sarcoglycan gene. Genetic analysis of one family has demonstrated linkage to another region on chromosome 18p; this gene has yet to be identified.

Onset is typically in the first or second decade. Myoclonus is the most prominent feature, primarily affecting the arms, shoulders, neck, and trunk and less commonly affecting the face and legs. The myoclonic jerks can be triggered by voluntary movements (action myoclonus) and are particularly evident as overflow jerks (i.e., involving body regions not involved in the action per se). The myoclonic component may respond to alcohol. Dystonia, usually torticollis and/or writer's cramp, occurs in some but not all affected patients and rarely is the only symptom of the disease. Psychiatric abnormalities, including panic attacks and obsessive–compulsive behavior, are frequently observed.

RPD (DYT12)

RPD is a rare autosomal-dominant disorder characterized by the rapid onset (or marked worsening) of dystonia and parkinsonism, usually over hours or days, which then plateaus. Linkage analysis in the affected families points to a defect on the long arm of chromosome 19 and the gene which codes for Na/K+ ATPase alpha 3 has been identified. This disorder commonly starts in adolescence. The dystonia can be focal, segmental, or generalized. Dysarthria, grimacing, bradykinesia, postural instability, and psychiatric disturbances are also described. There is little response to therapy, including dopaminergics and anticholinergics.

Paroxysmal Dyskinesias

The inherited paroxysmal dyskinesias, associated with gene loci DYT8 and DYT10, differ from the above-described genetic dystonias insofar as the dystonic features are clinically transient. The pathogenesic mechanisms that underlie these fluctuating disorders await further clarification, but the PNKD gene, myofibrillogeneses regulator, was recently identified.

Paroxysmal nonkinesigenic dystonia/dyskinesia (PNKD)

PNKD is an autosomal-dominant disorder. As its name implies, it is characterized by paroxysms of hyperkinesias, which can include dystonia, dyskinesia, choreoathetosis, and ballism. The paroxysms are not triggered by volitional movements, but may be precipitated by various factors such as stress and alcohol. Age of onset varies from infancy to adulthood, with adolescence being most common. The attacks may occur several times a day and last from minutes to hours.

Paroxysmal kinesigenic dystonia/dyskinesia (PKD)

PKD is also autosomal dominant, though sporadic cases have been reported. There is likely significant variable expressivity, with an apparent male predominance. Tomita and colleagues studied several affected Japanese families in 1999 and mapped the disease locus to chromosome 16. Different loci on chromosome 16 may be responsible in other affected families. Age of onset is generally during childhood. Seizures have been associated with the disorder and may begin in infancy. The paroxysms, unlike those in PNKD, are triggered by sudden movement, are usually short—lasting less than a few minutes, and can occur hundreds of times each day. PKD often responds well to anticonvulsant medication. Table 2.4 summarizes the salient differences between PNKD and PKD.

TABLE 2.4	**Features of Paroxysmal Nonkinesigenic Dystonia/Dyskinesia (PNKD) and Paroxysmal Kinesigenic Dystonia/Dyskinesia (PKD)**	
	PNKD	**PKD**
Chromosome	2	16
Mode of inheritance	AD	AD
Age of onset	Adolescence	Childhood
Triggers	Coffee, alcohol, fatigue	Movements
Frequency of attacks	Daily	Hundreds/day
Associated features	—	Infantile seizures
Response to AEDs	—	Carbamazepine

AD=autosomal dominant; AED= antiepileptic drugs.

CASE 3

DG had a normal delivery and psychomotor development until the age of 6 months, when she experienced the first of 3 generalized tonic–clonic seizures for which she was started on phenobarbital. She was on phenobarbital until the age of 2 and had not experienced any seizures since. Starting at the age of 8 years, she was noted to have recurrent episodes of involuntary limb movements when running to the mailbox. These movements, described as "arm extensions and toe curling," would last for 30 seconds. At times during these paroxysmal episodes she might not be able to speak, but retained full consciousness. There was no postictal period and no loss of bowel or bladder control. After examination by a pediatric neurologist, with negative results on electroencephalogram and MRI, she was finally diagnosed as having PKD. She was again started on phenobarbital, but this medication caused depression and had to be suspended. Her therapy was changed to Tegretol (carbamazepine) 100 mg/day, which successfully prevented further episodes. When she reached puberty at the age of 12, the Tegretol was increased to a twice-a-day dosing. Most recently, she was taking Tegretol-XR 200 mg once a day. She noticed that if she missed more than 1 dose, she experienced paroxysmal dystonic episodes. She believed that her episodes were now stronger and could occur more frequently. If unmedicated, she could have as many as 10 episodes per day.

SUMMARY

The distinctive features of the various primary dystonias are becoming increasingly clear as the genetic understanding behind them emerges. For the clinician, sorting out these entities can be a great challenge. By evaluating the age of onset and the body regions affected with the dystonia, as well as concomitant neurologic findings, differential and diagnostic plans can be formulated. With the increasing availability of genetic testing, a definitive diagnosis for some forms of dystonia can now be made. Because DYT1 dystonia is caused by the same recurring mutation in all patients, testing is relatively straightforward and commercially available. For DRD and myoclonus dystonia, it is necessary to screen for multiple different mutations, and at present, there are only a handful of laboratories that will perform this screening. It is important to provide genetic counseling when performing these genetic tests because the implications of both positive and negative tests need to be explained. For example, even if the test is negative, a genetic etiology is not excluded and this needs to be discussed. If the test is positive, a diagnosis is secured, but this diagnosis impacts on other at-risk family members. Also, the psychologic and social implications of a disorder with autosomal-dominant inheritance that has markedly reduced penetrance and very variable expression are complex and usually require in-depth discussion.

Most important, of course, are the corollary advances in therapy that may be the result of our continuing genetic insights. Recently developed cellular and animal models are helping in our understanding of the mechanisms that lead to dystonia. These comprise one of the many promising advances helping to unravel the mechanisms causing dystonia and providing a key to successful treatment and a cure.

ADDITIONAL READING

Up-to-date information on genetic counseling and testing can be obtained at http://www.geneclinics.org.

Almasy L, Bressman SB, Raymond D, Kramer PL, Greene PE, Heiman GA, et al. Idiopathic torsion dystonia linked to chromosome 8 in two Mennonite families. *Ann Neurol* 1997;42:670–673.

Brashear A, Butler IJ, Ozelius LJ, Kramer IP, Farlow MR, Breakefield XO, et al. Rapid-onset dystonia-parkinsonism: a report of clinical, biochemical, and genetic studies in two families. *Adv Neurol* 1998b;78:335–340.

Bressman SB, Sabatti C, Raymond D, et al. The DYT1 phenotype and guidelines for diagnostic testing. *Neurology* 2000;54:1746–1752.

Caldwell GA, Cao S, Sexton EG, Gelwix CC, Bevel JP, Caldwell KA. Suppression of polyglutamine-induced protein aggregation in Caenorhabditis elegans by torsin proteins. *Hum Mol Genet* 2003;12:307–319.

Cif L, El Fertit H, Vayssiere N, Hemm S, Hardouin E, Gannau A, et al. Treatment of dystonic syndromes by chronic electrical stimulation of the internal globus pallidus. *J Neurosurg Sci* 2003;47:52–55.

deCarvalho Aquiar P, Sweadner KJ, Penniston JT, Zaremba J, Lui L, Canton M, et al. Mutations in the Na+/K+ ATPase alpha 3 gene ATP1A3 are associated with rapid-onset dystonia parkinsonism. *Neuron* 2004;43:169–173.

Dobyns WB, Ozelius LJ, Kramer PL, Brashear A, Farlow MR, Perry TR, et al. Rapid-onset dystonia-Parkinson's. *Neurology* 1993;43:2596–2602.

Fahn S, Marsden CD, Calne DB. Classification and investigation in dystonia. In: Marsden CD, Fahn S, (eds.) *Movement Disorders 2*. London: Butterworth and Co.; 1987:332–358.

Gasser T. Inherited myoclonus-dystonia syndrome. *Adv Neurol* 1998; 78:325–334.

Grimes DA, Han F, Lang AE, St George-Hyssop P, Racacho L, Bulman DE. A novel locus for inherited myoclonus-dystonia on 18p11. *Neurology* 2002;59:1183–1186.

Hewett J, Gonzalez-Agosti C, Slater D, Ziefer P, Li S, Bergeron D, et al. Mutant torsinA, responsible for early-onset torsion dystonia, forms membrane inclusions in cultured neural cells. *Hum Mol Genet* 2000;9:1403–1413.

Ichinose H, Nagatsu T, Sumi-Ichinose C, Nimura T. Dopa-responsive dystonia. In: Pulst S, (ed.) *Genetics of Movement Disorders*. San Diego: Academic Press; 2002:419–428.

Klein C, Breakfield XO, Ozelius L. Genetics of primary dystonia. *Semin Neurol* 1999;19:271–280.

Klein C, Friedman J, Bressman S, Vieregge P, Brin MF, Pramstaller PP, et al. Genetic testing for early-onset torsion dystonia (DYT1): introduction of a simple screening method, experiences from testing of a large patient cohort, and ethical aspects. *Genet Test* 1999;3:323–328.

Knappskog PM, Flatmark T, Mallet J, Ludecke B, Bartholome K. Recessively inherited L-DOPA-responsive dystonia caused by a point mutation (Q381K) in the tyrosine hydroxylase gene. *Hum Mol Genet* 1995;4:1209–1212.

Kramer PL, de Leon D, Ozelius LJ, Risch NJ, Bressman SB, Brin MF, et al. Dystonia gene in Ashkenazi Jewish population is located on chromosome 9q32-34. *Ann Neurol* 1990;27:114–120.

Lance JW. Familial paroxysmal dystonic choreoathetosis and its differentiation from related syndromes. *Ann Neurol* 1977;2: 285–293.

Leube B, Hendgen T, Kessler KR, Knapp M, Benecke R, Auburger G. Sporadic focal dystonia in Northwest Germany: molecular basis on chromosome 18p. *Ann Neurol* 1997;42:111–114.

McNaught KS, Kapustin A, Jackson T, Jengelley TA, Inobaptiste R, Shashidharan P, et al. Brainstem pathology in DYT1 primary dystonia. *Ann Neurol* 2004;56:540–547.

Muller U. Primary Dystonias. In: Pulst S, (ed.) *Genetics of Movement Disorders*. San Diego: Academic Press, 2002;395–418.

Nemeth A. The genetics of primary dystonias and related disorders. *Brain* 2000;125:695–721.

Ozelius L, Bressman SB. DYT1 dystonia. In: Pulst S, (ed.) *Genetics of Movement Disorders*. San Diego: Academic Press; 2002:407–415.

Ozelius LJ, Hewett JW, Page CE, Bressman SB, Kramer PL, Shalish C, de Leon D, Klein C, et al. The early-onset torsion dystonia gene (DYT1) encodes an ATP-binding protein. *Nat Genet* 1997;17:40–48.

Ozelius L, Kramer PL, Moskowitz CB, Kwiatkowski DJ, Brin MF, Bressman SB, et al. Human gene for torsion dystonia located on chromosome 9q32-q34. *Neuron* 1989;2:1427–1434.

Rainer S, Thomas D, Tokarz D, Ming L, Bui M, Plein E, et al. Myofibrillogenesis regulator/gene mutations cause paroxysmal dystonic choreoathetogis. *Arch Neuro* 2004;61:1025–1029.

Shang H, Clerc N, Lang D, Kaelin-Lang A, Burgunder JM. Clinical and molecular genetic evaluation of patients with primary dystonis. *Eur J Neurol* 2005;12(2):131–138.

Tagliati M, Alterman RL, Shils JL, Miravite J, Bressman SB. Progressive improvement of generalized dystonia after pallidal deep brain stimulation. *Neurology* 2003;60(suppl 1):A344.

Tomita H-A, Nagamitsu S, Wakui K, Fukushima Y, Yamada K, Sadamatsu M, et al. Paroxysmal Kinesigenic Choreoathetosis locus maps to chromosome 16p11.2-q12.1. *Am J Hum Genet* 1999;65:1688–1697.

Valente EM, Bentivoglio AR, Cassetta E, Dixon PH, Davis MB, Ferraris A, et al. DYT13, a novel primary torsion dystonia locus, maps to chromosome 1p36.13-36.32 in an Italian family with cranial-cervical or upper limb onset. *Ann Neurol* 2001;49:662–666.

Walker RH, Brin MF, Sandu D, Good PF, Shashidharan P. TorsinA immunoreactivity in brains of patients with DYT1 and non-DYT1 dystonia. *Neurology* 2002;58:120–124.

Yianni J, Bain PG, Gregory RP, Nandi D, Joint C, Scott RB, et al. Postoperative progress of dystonia patients following globus pallidus internus deep brain stimulation. *Eur J Neurol* 2003;10:239–247.

Zimprich A, Grabowski M, Asmus F, Naumann M, Berg D, Bertram M, et al. Mutations in the gene encoding epsilon-sarcoglycan cause myoclonus-dystonia syndrome. *Nat Genet* 2001;29:66–69.

CHAPTER 3

CRANIOCERVICAL DYSTONIA

Joseph K.C. Tsui, MBBS, MRCP, FRCP(C)

CASE 1

A 50-year-old man presented at a movement disorders clinic with a history of frequent involuntary eyelid blinking for about 6 months. His eyes had been feeling gritty for some time, and he had to blink hard to relieve the discomfort. He was seen previously by an ophthalmologist, who told him that his eyes were normal. Some eyedrops were prescribed, but he did not find them helpful. The symptoms became worse over the past 6 months in that blinking occurred now so frequently that reading was affected. Examination of the patient revealed no specific abnormalities except for frequent involuntary blinking, sometimes associated with facial grimacing.

It is likely that this patient has a form of adult-onset focal dystonia known as *blepharospasm*. This is the second most common form of focal dystonia (in this case, cranial dystonia), and diagnosis is made by exclusion. An ophthalmologic examination to rule out local eye pathology is important when in doubt. The onset is usually insidious, presenting with irritation of the eyes associated with frequent blinking. Initially, symptoms may be unilateral or asymmetric, but given time, bilateral involvement is the rule. Severity may range from mild (requiring no treatment) to severe (eyes shut most of the day to the point that some may register as legally blind). In some cases, dystonia may spread to involve the lower face and jaws; this combination is sometimes known as Meige's syndrome. Some important differential diagnoses include tics, hemifacial spasm, myasthenia gravis, and eyelid-opening apraxia.

The etiology is unknown. When cranial dystonia occurs as a part of generalized dystonia (idiopathic torsion dystonia), there may be an association with the DYT1 gene. Of these patients, 1/3 may have a family history of hand tremor or other forms of focal dystonia. In most cases, however, family history is negative. In the majority of cases, no pathology in the nervous system can be found. It is suggestive that the biochemical pathology may lie in the basal ganglia or upper brainstem.

Treatment options include oral medications, botulinum toxin injections, and surgery. A long list of oral medications has been reported to be helpful in some cases of blepharospasm including:

- Anticholinergic drugs
- Baclofen
- Levodopa or other dopaminergics
- Dopamine receptor blockers
- Dopamine depletors
- Benzodiazepines
- Carbamazepines

Effects are usually unsatisfactory and side effects from these drugs are not easily tolerated because some would need to be administered at high doses.

Surgical treatment includes myectomy (removal of part of the orbicularis oculi), blepharoplasty, and selective denervation of the orbicularis oculi. Results of these treatments are usually inconsistent.

TREATMENT WITH BOTULINUM TOXIN INJECTIONS

Botulinum toxin (BoNT) is a food poison, produced by *Clostridium botulinum*. It is a protein with at least 7 antigenic types: A, B, C1/C2, D, E, F, and G. Only types A, B, and F cause botulism in humans. These serotypes are different in their potency, and species difference is tremendous. BoNT produces a presynaptic neuromuscular blockade, preventing the release of acetylcholine. It consists of a heavy chain and a light chain. The former is important in binding to the presynaptic neuromuscular terminals, whereas the latter is released into the terminals. The light chain is a zinc metalloendopeptidase, which cleaves the vesicle-docking protein complex important in the process of exocytosis and acetylcholine release. The nerve terminal reacts by sprouting new extensions, which would recede once new connections are made with the motor end plates. This process takes approximately 3 months for type A toxin, which explains the duration of action. Type A toxin was the earliest to be used in humans (Botox®; Allergan, Irvine, CA and Dysport®; Ipsen, Slough, Berkshire, UK). Another serotype, B, is also available

(Myobloc™; Solstice Neurosciences, San Diego, CA). BoNT is a biologic substance quantified in terms of the mouse unit (MU), a biologic unit representing the LD50 for a standard strain of mice with a standard weight.

BoNT has become the treatment of choice in the past 2 decades. Local intramuscular injections of BoNT into the orbicularis oculi muscles may provide symptomatic improvement for about 3 months, when the treatment would need to be repeated. Side effects include local bruises following injection, ptosis, visual blurring, diplopia, dry eyes, and sometimes droopiness of the angle of the mouth. These are usually transient and self-limiting. Patients may receive trimonthly injections indefinitely without any significant long-term adverse effects.

CASE 2

While attending a regular repeat BoNT previously discussed injection session, the patient brought along his 43-year-old sister, who was noted to have involuntary head turning to the left. The onset was insidious, beginning with some soreness in her neck 2 years ago. This gradually evolved to more severe pain on the left side of her neck. A year ago, her head started to turn to the left involuntarily. This was initially intermittent and did not affect her daily activities, but in the last 6 months has become more persistent. She has to give up working as a secretary, and she finds that she is unable to keep her eyes on the road when she is driving because of the head turning movements, and shoulder checking to her right is not possible.

The most likely diagnosis in this case is cervical dystonia (CD). This condition is the most common form of adult-onset focal dystonia, with peak incidence during the fifth decade. There is a slight female preponderance of approximately 1.7:1. The onset is usually insidious, characterized by involuntary head and neck deviation with abnormal posturing. Pain is a common feature, occurring in over 70% of cases. Superimposed on the sustained abnormal posturing may be fast or slow jerky movements that may be involuntary or corrective, and tremulous movements may be present.

The diagnosis is usually made on clinical grounds, based on characteristic clinical features and exclusion of secondary causes of a twisted neck. There are no laboratory or radiological tests for confirmation.

This patient had been seen by several physicians, but no firm diagnosis was provided. She was referred to a psychiatrist, who started her on antidepressants, but the drugs only produced fatigue. The symptoms were most bothersome during certain activities, such as driving, sitting in the dentist's or the hairdresser's chair, or working at the computer. Walking improved her symptoms; touching her chin with her fingers offered her temporary relief of the head and neck movements. Left-sided neck pain was aggravated by sitting for any length of time, and she experienced occipital headaches when the neck pain became more severe. Her neck felt completely relaxed upon awakening in the morning, but within minutes of waking up, it would begin to twist.

It is common for a patient with CD to remain undiagnosed for variable periods of time. This condition was previously thought to be of psychogenic origin, and frequently patients would be given antidepressants or psychotropic drugs.

Dystonic movements typically fluctuate in severity according to a patient's activities. Some may find sitting better than standing, and vice versa. Self-applied sensory stimuli may improve head and neck movements, as described in this patient. This phenomenon is known as "sensory trick," or geste antagoniste. As a rule, dystonia subsides when the patient is sleeping.

This patient's past health had been good, with no major illnesses or operations. She was married, with an 8-year-old son who was doing well at school. Her husband, a salesman, was very supportive. There was no similar family history. Her maternal uncle, 67 years of age, had recently been diagnosed with Parkinson's disease. She does not smoke and does not drink alcohol, and there is no history of recreational drug abuse.

Most patients do not have any significant underlying medical illnesses, and the onset is unprovoked, though some may experience an acute precipitation of symptoms following minor head or neck injury or surgery that may or may not have been related to the neck. Family history of CD is uncommon, in the region of 5% to 8%. However, family history of other forms of focal dystonia, such as writer's cramp or blepharospasm, may be detected on more detailed and repeated questioning during subsequent visits, and up to 25% may have a relative with some form of dystonia. This condition is not related to Parkinson's disease. In some patients, the presentation may be predominantly head tremor with relatively little neck twisting, and the possibility of Parkinson's disease is sometimes considered during the workup of the patient.

Examination revealed that the patient had persistent head turning to the left when sitting. Intermittent movements were present when trying to return the head to central position. Her right sternocleidomastoid appeared hypertrophic. The muscles of the left side of the neck appeared very active, and were tender on deep palpation. The left shoulder was elevated and displaced forward. Range of movement was normal to the left, but the patient could barely turn her head just past the midline to the right. Head tremor was present when she tried to maintain her head looking to the right. The rest of the neurologic examination was normal.

The above describes a typical result of physical examination of CD. The neurologic examination should be normal apart from the abnormal head and neck findings. Hypertrophy of neck muscles is a common feature, the sternocleidomastoid muscle contralateral to the side of turning being most frequently described because it is most visible. Shoulder elevation is another common finding, and the muscle involved is usually the ipsilateral levator scapulae rather than the trapezius.

Neck x-rays showed mild degenerative changes in this patient's cervical spine. Computed tomography scan of her head was normal. Laboratory reports on her complete blood count, electrolytes, and renal and liver functions were all normal.

In most cases, only x-rays of the neck would be necessary to rule out structural lesions of the cervical spine. Differential diagnoses include the following:

1. Structural lesions of the vertebrae, such as congenital abnormalities, fracture, or dislocation.
2. Drug-induced dystonia. Dopamine-receptor blockers (neuroleptic drugs) may cause any kind of movement disorders, including dystonia. It is, however, uncommon to present with neck dystonia alone. It may be present in association with tardive orofacial dyskinesia or parkinsonism. In such cases, the more common pattern is retrocollis.
3. Ocular torticollis. A cranial nerve (CN) IV palsy with weakness of the superior oblique muscle may lead to diplopia, corrected by tilting the head to the ipsilateral side. This is uncommon, and head tilting usually begins in childhood.
4. Sandifer syndrome. This is a pediatric condition, with the child tilting the head to the left to relieve discomfort related to hiatus hernia.
5. Psychogenic torticollis. This is actually uncommon, and is diagnosed by exclusion.
6. Other rarer possibilities include Arnold-Chiari malformation and posterior fossa tumor. Association with a tilted neck has been reported in these conditions.

After reviewing the investigation results, the patient was anxious to learn the nature and prognosis of her condition. She raised the question whether this condition is inheritable, since her 8-year-old son lately seemed to be experiencing intermittent, though infrequent, jerky movements of his neck.

The etiology of CD is unknown. It is believed to be related to circuitary abnormalities in the basal ganglia, resulting in imbalance of nervous impulses to the neck muscles. In most postmortem series, no consistent pathologic findings were found. In generalized dystonia (idiopathic torsion dystonia), DYT1—a gene that encodes for TorsinA—has been found to be responsible in many families. However, in CD, only 1 family in Germany has been described to present with craniocervical dystonia (in this family, DYT7 has been proposed as the responsible gene); the majority of cases are sporadic. In addition, CD presents typically in adult life. It is therefore unlikely that her child would develop cervical dystonia. He might actually have simple tics, which is not related to dystonia.

The patient asked what could be done for her.

Since the cause of this condition is unknown, no cure is available. Only symptomatic therapy can be offered. Options include oral medications, botulinum toxin injections, and surgery. Supportive therapy such as physiotherapy, occupational therapy, and stress management are important aspects of treatment.

TREATMENT WITH ORAL MEDICATIONS
The treatment of dystonia historically has been based on oral medications, which may provide partial symptomatic relief in some cases.

Anticholinergic agents have been the best evaluated of all the oral medications. These are represented by trihexyphenidyl and benztropine. It has been estimated that these drugs are effective in over 40% of patients with generalized dystonia, but much less successful in adult-onset focal dystonia, including CD. High doses, which are better tolerated by children, are necessary to produce results. This treatment is limited by side effects such as dry mouth, blurred vision, urinary retention in prostatism, precipitation of glaucoma, and confusion and hallucinations with higher doses.

Baclofen has been effective in up to 20% of patients with dystonia, again mostly in children. Intrathecal baclofen is less useful in CD since this concentration drops approximately 4-fold by the time it reaches the cervical region from the lumbar site of introduction.

Benzodiazepines, including clonazepam, has been effective in approximately 15% of patients, but tolerance is common. Lorazepam may attenuate the severity of symptoms simply by reducing the level of anxiety, which is a general relieving factor for CD. *Antidepressants* are sometimes used based on similar principles.

Levodopa preparations, though producing dramatic responses in patients with dopa-responsive dystonia, are rarely useful in the management of adult-onset CD. Likewise, dopamine agonists are not expected to be effective in CD. *Dopamine receptor–blocking agents* or *dopamine–depleting agents* are more likely to offer symptomatic relief in some patients. In general, the latter are preferred because they are unlikely to initiate drug-induced movement disorders. Tetrabenazine, being predominantly a presynaptic dopamine-depleting agent, may be tried in some patients.

Other drugs such as *anticonvulsants* (carbamazepine) have been effective in individual cases.

In summary, oral medications yield unpredictable and disappointing results in CD, and BoNT injections have become the treatment of choice in many centers.

TREATMENT WITH BoNT INJECTIONS

BoNT injections offer symptomatic improvement for CD patients, lasting approximately 3 months per treatment. It is now generally believed that "booster" doses (re-injections 2 to 4 weeks after a treatment) should not be performed because of the potential possibility of immunizing the patient against BoNT.

Side effects from BoNT injections may be divided into 4 categories: generalized, local, undesirable muscle weakness, and immune reactions. Patients may report generalized discomfort such as fatigue, malaise, headaches, dizziness, nausea, and flu-like symptoms. All these are transient and resolve spontaneously within a few days. In a published double-blind study, more patients complained of these generalized side effects when they received placebo injections. Local pain and ecchymoses around the injection site may occur. Local trauma may be minimized by using small-gauged needles, such as 30 G, and by avoiding injecting a large volume into a single site. Neck weakness may occur in some patients who are unusually sensitive to the injections. Dysphagia has been reported to occur in 1.7% to 90% of patients, and is believed to be related to local diffusion of BoNT into the pharyngeal muscles. It has been suggested that bilateral sternocleidomastoid injections are more prone to producing dysphagia, but this has not been found to be a factor in some centers. Allergic reactions have not been clearly documented in CD

patients receiving BoNT injections. Dry mouth appears to be a common side effect of Myobloc.

SURGICAL TREATMENT

Bilateral Anterior Cervical Rhizotomy
Before 1960, this was the standard procedure for CD. Denervation is limited downward to a portion of CN IV because of the phrenic nerve, and cannot be extended to all the posterior cervical muscles involved. Many experience neck weakness and limitation of voluntary movements. This procedure has lost popularity now.

Epidural Cervical Stimulation
In one report, this procedure was described as producing marked improvement in over 37% of patients. However, another report did not find any objective evidence of improvement in CD.

Microvascular Lysis of the Accessory Nerve Roots
The basis of this procedure has not been well founded since the accessory nerve roots supply only a portion of neck muscles responsible for CD.

Myectomy
Extensive resection of muscles may be required in most instances, but selective peripheral denervation is apparently a more accepted procedure, although based on very similar principles of knocking out excessive muscular activities.

Selective Peripheral Denervation
The objective is to denervate all the muscles involved in the abnormal head and neck movements while sparing other muscles to preserve normal voluntary movements of the neck. This is a lengthy procedure, requiring identification and confirmation of the muscles to be denervated by individual stimulation. Also known as the "Bertrand procedure," this surgery is described as working best for rotational torticollis and shoulder elevation. Antecollis remains difficult to treat.

SUPPORTIVE TREATMENTS

Nursing
The nurse can explain and reinforce information given to patients by physicians and relieve frustration and anger that patients and family members have suffered before being referred to a movement disorder clinic. A specially trained nurse can spend more time with a patient than a physician can afford to and can help to advise patients to initiate oral medications, thereby saving many unnecessary phone calls.

Physical Therapy

Activities and exercises may be important in day-to-day management of many patients with CD. They should be advised that they have overactivity in the neck muscles, and not weakness. After BoNT injections, the injected muscles should be stretched, rather than exercised, to build them up again. A soft collar can be made to size for individual patients. This is better than a hard, stiff collar, which may cause abrasions as a result of excessive neck movements inside the neck brace.

Occupational Therapy

Yet another important aspect of supportive management for CD, occupational therapy helps to promote, maintain, and restore occupational performance, health, and well being.

Other important aspects of treatment include *stress management* and *psychiatric referral* for those with secondary depression and anxiety.

The patient decided on treatment with BoNT injections, and responded very well. After 6 months, during which she underwent treatment sessions, she was able to return to work as a part-time secretary. Approximately 3 to 4 days following each treatment, her symptoms improved. The effects would begin to wear off by about 10 weeks; she returned for repeat treatment at the end of 12 weeks. She remained stable for 2 years, until a motor vehicle accident in which she sustained a whiplash injury. She had severe neck pain following the injury and felt that the BoNT injections were not as effective as before.

This brings on the complicated issue of posttraumatic CD. In some patients, the onset of symptoms may relate to minor head or neck injuries. Whether posttraumatic CD is a separate entity from idiopathic CD is controversial. Clinical features in this group of patients appear to be different: There is more prominent pain aggravated by any head movements; the head and neck are more fixed, with extreme limitations in range of movements; and the "sensory trick" phenomenon is absent. The abnormal posture persists through sleep. In these cases, the response to BoNT injections is usually poor. Patients who have idiopathic CD, and who incur exacerbation of symptoms following injury, may find BoNT injections not very helpful because pain in such cases is difficult to control. They may need more analgesics and muscle relaxants as adjunctive therapy.

ADDITIONAL READING

Bressman SB. Dystonia genotypes, phenotypes, and classification. *Adv Neurol* 2004;94:101–107.

Callahan A. Blepharospasm with resection of part of orbicularis nerve supply. *Arch Ophthalmol* 1963;70:508–511.

Cardoso F, Jankovic J. Blepharospasm. In: Tsui JK, Calne DB, (eds.) *Handbook of Dystonia*. New York: Marcel Dekker Inc.; 1995:129–141.

Chan J, Brin MF, Fahn S. Idiopathic CD: clinical characteristics. *Mov Disord* 1991;6:119–126.

Comella CL, Jankovic J, Brin MF. Use of botulinum toxin type A in the treatment of cervical dystonia. *Neurology* 2000;55(12 suppl 5):S15–S21.

Dutton JJ, Buckley EG. Botulinum toxin in the management of blepharospasm. *Arch Neurol* 1986;43:380–382.

Jankovic J, Ford J. Blepharospasm and orofacial-cervical dystonia: clinical and pharmacological findings in 100 patients. *Ann Neurol* 1983;13:402–411.

Jankovic J, Nutt JG. Blepharospasm and cranial-cervical dystonia (Meige's syndrome): familial occurrence. In: Jankovic J, Tolosa E, (eds.) *Advances in Neurology*. 49: Facial Dyskinesias. New York: Raven Press; 1988:117–123.

Leube B, Hendgen T, Kessler KR, Knapp M, Benecke R, Auburger G. Evidence of DYT7 being a common cause of cervical dystonia (torticollis) in Central Europe. *Am J Med Genet* 1997;74:529–532.

McCord CD, Shore JW, Putnam JR. Treatment of essential blepharospasm: II. A modification of exposure of the muscle stripping technique. *Arch Ophthalmol* 1984;102:269–273.

Ozelius LJ, Hewett JW, Page CE, et al. The gene (DYT1) for early-onset torsion dystonia encodes a novel protein related to the Clp protease/heat shock family. *Adv Neurol* 1998;78:93–105.

Tarsy D. Comparison of acute- and delayed-onset posttraumatic cervical dystonia. *Mov Disord* 1998;13(3):481–485.

Tsui JK, Eisen A, Stoessl AJ, Calne S, Calne DB. Double-blind study of botulinum toxin in spasmodic torticollis. *Lancet* 1986;2:245–247.

Waddy HM, Fletcher NA, Harding AE, Marsden CD. A genetic study of idiopathic focal dystonias. *Ann Neurol* 1991;29:320–324.

CHAPTER 4

LIMB AND GENERALIZED DYSTONIA

Mark A. Stacy, MD

INTRODUCTION

Dystonia consists of sustained, repetitive, patterned contractions of muscles that produce twisting (e.g., torticollis) or squeezing (e.g., blepharospasm) movements or abnormal postures that may be present at rest, with changing posture, or when performing a specific motor activity. Oppenheimer coined the term "dystonia muscularum deformans" in 1911 to describe a group of children with abnormal postures and progressive disability. However, because dystonia is not a disorder of muscle, and does not produce postural deformity, the shortened term is now preferred. Over the last 90 years, the classification of this disorder has evolved from clinical characterizations—such as focal, segmental, or generalized dystonia—to molecular descriptions describing a number of alleles associated with these conditions. Increasingly, careful phenotypic analyses within specific kindreds have led to the realization that a wide range of clinical presentations may exist within a specific genotype. The first of these genetic characterizations, DYT1, is an autosomal-dominant disorder localized to chromosome 9q32-34. This population represents the dystonia musculorum deformans subjects originally described by Oppenheimer.

EPIDEMIOLOGY

Although population studies may underestimate actual disease frequencies, reported rates of dystonia vary from 127 to 329 per 1 million. One practice-based epidemiologic study from a large clinic in Munich, Germany resulted in the diagnosis of primary dystonia in 188 of 230 referral subjects. These data suggest point prevalence ratios of 101 per 1 million for focal and 30 per 1 million for generalized primary dystonia. The Epidemiologic Study of Dystonia in Europe Collaborative Group has also completed an epidemiologic review of dystonia. In this investigation of the relative frequencies of 957 subjects with primary dystonia, limb dystonia was seen in 109 subjects (15.0%), while segmental, multifocal, and generalized dystonia was seen in 200 subjects (20.9%), 17 (1.8%), and 12 (1.3%), respectively. There were no differences related to gender in the limb dystonia group, and the mean age of onset was 34.4 years for women and 41.7 years for men. Women were almost twice as likely to be diagnosed with segmental dystonia when compared with men.

CLINICAL PRESENTATION

Dystonia may be primary or secondary in etiology. The primary dystonias are often associated with genetic changes and are now grouped under the term "primary torsion dystonia." Familial and population studies of allele carriers demonstrate a wide range of symptoms ranging from generalized (affecting the entire body) to focal (confined to one body part). Focal dystonias involve the head (cranial dystonia), neck (cervical dystonia), or limb. The most common form of limb dystonia is writer's cramp, a task-specific dystonia. The presentation of a subject with idiopathic dystonia is highly variable, usually begins as a focal dystonia of the legs, and is initially present with action, such as walking. In adult-onset limb dystonia, the dystonia usually remains confined to the originally affected location. However, an initial presentation in a patient younger than age 18 or with bilateral lower extremity onset is usually associated with progression to generalized dystonia.

Limb dystonia consists of sustained, repetitive, and patterned contractions of muscles that produce an abnormal posture of the upper or lower limb that may be present at rest, when changing position, or when performing a specific motor activity. Focal, segmental, and generalized dystonic disorders may produce symptoms of limb dystonia. Involvement of the upper extremity is most often associated with "writer's cramp," a task-specific, focal dystonia, but may evolve from being only an activity-related abnormality to, at its most severe, being present at rest.

Writer's cramp postures may produce any combination of finger flexion or extension, wrist flexion or extension, and elbow flexion. Patients with extensor muscle involvement notice difficulty putting the pen on paper, the thumb or fingers lifting off the pen, and a need to lean further and further toward the writing surface to compensate for wrist extension. In this instance a faint script with broad loops may be noted, since the patient has difficulty maintaining contact between the pen and paper (Figure 4.1).

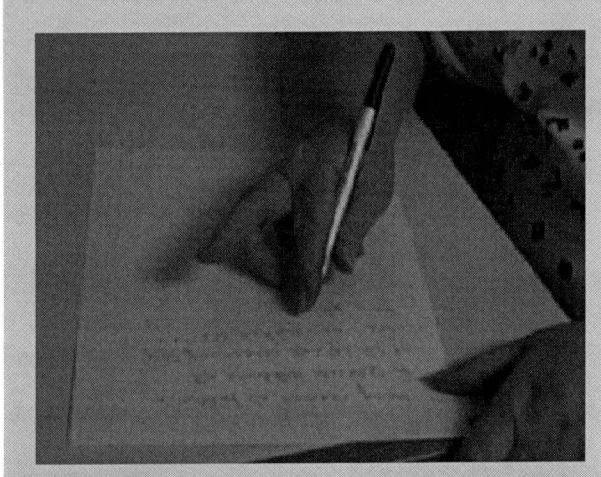

FIGURE 4.1 This 36-year-old accountant with 3-year history of progressive hand cramping and writing difficulty underwent 10 injection sessions, and now receives only 7 units botulinum toxin type A to the extensor digitorum complex.

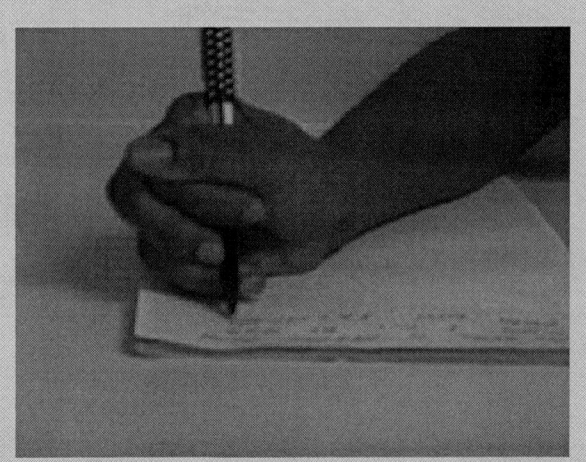

FIGURE 4.2 This 15-year-old girl was referred to a psychologist for poor school performance attributed to defiance because she would not complete her writing assignments. She was diagnosed with writer's cramp and became successful with minor modification of her in-class work and the use of a home computer to complete her assignments.

Conversely, a flexor-type writer's cramp will produce bold and illegible script. Flexion of the fingers decreases space between letters and loops, while wrist flexion increases the boldness of the script. In either situation, patients may adopt a printing style of handwriting, perhaps to allow for each letter to become a discreet component, instead of using more prolonged sequences of activity (Figure 4.2).

"Occupational dystonia" is a term used to describe patients with dystonic muscle contractions that result in employment disability. Occupations most often associated with these disorders are associated with chronic, stereotyped movements of the hands and fingers. Typists, stenographers, musicians, blackjack dealers, dentists, and surgeons have been reported to have this condition. Similar sports-related dystonias have also been reported in trapshooters, dartsmen, and golfers. The sudden jerklike movement of the extensor muscles of the lead forearm, while moving the club toward the ball when putting, is, in golfer's terminology, the "yips."

Limb dystonia involving the legs usually produces knee extension, plantar flexion, and toe flexion, but may involve any leg muscle. A common secondary cause of leg dystonia includes extension of the great toe ("Babinski dystonia") secondary to an ischemic lesion in the basal ganglia (usually putamen) (Figure 4.3).

Leg dystonia in patients beyond 30 years of age should prompt a concern for idiopathic Parkinson's disease. In children, the development of this posture may represent the initial onset of primary torsion dystonia or dopa-responsive dystonia.

DIFFERENTIAL DIAGNOSIS

There is increasing evidence that many adult-onset focal dystonias are genetically based. At this time, molecular descriptions of dystonic conditions have been reported with idiopathic torsion dystonia (DYT1), focal dystonias (DYT7), mixed dystonias (DYT6 and DYT13), dopa-responsive dystonia, myoclonic dystonia, rapid-onset dystonia parkinsonism, Fahr disease, Hallervorden–Spatz syndrome, X-linked dystonia parkinsonism, deafness–dystonia syndrome, mitochondrial dystonias, myoclonic dystonia, neuroacanthocytosis, and the paroxysmal dystonias/dyskinesias. In addition, focal dystonia may emerge in families exhibiting generalized dystonia and has also been related to the DYT1 allele (Table 4.1).

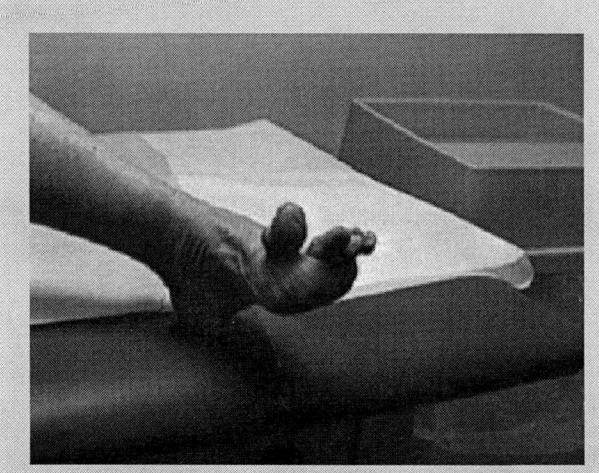

FIGURE 4.3 This 70-year-old woman with a history of mild hypertension had a small, left putamen infarction. She was hospitalized for mild weakness that resolved satisfactorily. Her workup was otherwise negative. Over the next 8 months she developed right great toe extension, toe abduction, and increased plantar arch. She responded to a botulinum toxin A injection of 50 units to the extensor hallucis longus muscle and 30 units to her flexor hallucis brevis muscle.

Extrapyramidal syndromes such as Wilson's disease, Parkinson's disease, progressive supranuclear palsy, corticobasal ganglionic degeneration, and multiple system atrophy may be associated with dystonia. Parkinson's disease may present with symptoms of lower limb dystonia. Patients with progressive supranuclear palsy often present with dystonic muscle contraction of the axial muscles, and some patients with corticobasal ganglionic degeneration will exhibit profound limb dystonia in addition to, and sometimes masking, symptoms of "alien-limb" phenomenon. Tonic spasms of multiple sclerosis are typically transient attacks of hemidystonia of the limbs. Reported secondary causes of dystonia include exposure to dopamine receptor–blocking drugs ("tardive dystonia") hypoxic encephalopathy, head trauma, encephalitis, human immunodeficiency virus (HIV) and other infections, peripheral or segmental nerve injury, reflex sympathetic dystrophy, inherited disorders (e.g., Wilson's disease), metabolic disorders and other inborn errors of metabolism, mitochondrial disorders, and chromosomal abnormalities (Table 4.2).

Central nervous system lesions are well recognized as causes of dystonia. In a review of 190 cases of hemidystonia, the most common etiologies of hemidystonia were stroke, trauma, and perinatal injury. In these subjects, the mean age of onset was 20 to 25.7 years, and the average latency from insult to dystonia was 2.8 to 4.1 years. Basal ganglia lesions were seen in almost 50% of patients, with the putamen most commonly involved. Cerebral infarction in the posterolateral thalamic nuclei may be associated with contralateral hand dystonia, and large lenticular or caudatocapsulolenticular lesions may give rise to foot dystonia. Other structural abnormalities associated with limb dystonia include cavernous angioma of the basal ganglia, subdural hematoma, left frontal meningioma, calcification of the head of the right caudate nucleus, and cervical cord lesion secondary to multiple sclerosis. Movement disorders after severe head injury have been reported in 13% to 66% of patients.

Although limb trauma as a cause of dystonia remains controversial, it has been suggested that pain, prominent in nearly all reported cases of posttraumatic dystonia, may be a critical pathogenic factor. Positron emission tomography increased blood flow in the basal ganglia is associated with painful thermal stimulation or capsaicin injection of the hand. This hypothesis is consistent with the observation that dystonia has resulted from electrical injury and soft tissue injury. However, there is a report of 4 patients who developed limb dystonia following casting for a fracture. Only 2 of these patients experienced pain during casting, which suggests that pain is not necessary and immobilization alone may be sufficient for the development of dystonia after peripheral injury.

In a review of 15 patients who developed cervical dystonia after head, neck, or shoulder trauma, 6 patients who exhibited symptoms of dystonia within 4 weeks of injury demonstrated reduced cervical mobility, prominent shoulder elevation, trapezius hypertrophy (in most of these patients), and the presence of sustained postures. This was strikingly similar to the situation of 2 additional patients described separately. In contrast, delayed onset of cervical dystonia was clinically indistinguishable from nontraumatic idiopathic cervical dystonia.

Psychogenic limb dystonia should be diagnosed only by exclusion and after thorough consideration of all other possibilities.

PATHOGENESIS AND PATHOPHYSIOLOGY

Writer's cramp is a task-specific dystonia that leads to involuntary hand postures during writing. Physiologically, coactivation of antagonistic groups of muscles in the upper limb muscles is seen during dystonic muscle activity, and antagonist muscle relaxation

TABLE 4.1 Clinical and Molecular Information on the Primary Dystonias

Locus/ Designation	Location	Inheritance Pattern	Phenotype	Testing Available
DYT1 ITD	9q34	AD (IP)	Childhood and adolescent; limb onset	Yes
DYT2	Unknown	AR	In Spanish Gypsies; not confirmed	No
DYT3	Xq13.1	XR	Parkinsonism-dystonia (Lubag, Philippines)	No
DYT4	Unknown	AD	Whispering dysphonia in Australian family	No
GCHI DYT5*	14q22	AD (IP)	Dopa-responsive dystonia	Research only
DYT6	8p21-p22	AD	Mennonite/Amish dystonia with mixed face/eyes/neck or limb onset; childhood or adult onset	No
DYT7 IFD	18p	AD (IP)	German families; adult neck, face, or limb onset	No
PNKD DYT8*	2q33-q35	AD (IP)	Paroxysmal dystonia or choreoathetosis	No
CSE DYT9*	1p	AD	Paroxysmal choreoathetosis with episodic ataxia and spasticity	No
PKC DYT10*	16p11.2-q12.1	AD (IP)	Paroxysmal kinesigenic choreoathetosis	No
SGCE DYT11*	7q21	AD (IP)	Myoclonic dystonia; alcohol responsive	Research?
DYT12	19q13	AD (IP)	Rapid-onset parkinsonism	No
DYT13	1p36.13-32	AD (IP)	Italian family; cranial or cervical dystonia	No
LDYT	Mt DNA		Leber's hereditary optic neuropathy	No
BGC1 Fahr's disease	14q	AD	Progressive dystonia, parkinsonism, dysphagia, ataxia	No
PANK2 Hallervorden-Spatz syndrome	20p12.3-p13	AR	Dystonia, parkinsonism, dementia, ocular abnormalities; childhood onset; "tiger eye" sign on MRI	Research only
PARK2	6q25.2-q27	AR	Juvenile-onset Parkinson's disease	Research only
XK McLeod Syndrome	Xp21	XR	Areflexia, dystonia, orofacial dyskinesias, tics, epilepsy, cardiomyopathy	Research only
CHAC Chorea-acanthocytosis	9q21	AR	Orofacial dyskinesia/mutilation, tics, limb dystonia, chorea, hyporeflexia, weakness, seizures, parkinsonism, dementia	Research only
DFN-1/MTS X-Linked deafness	Xq21.3-q22	XR	Sensorineural hearing loss, dystonia, optic atrophy, mental retardation, neuropathy	Research only

*Previous nomenclature; replaced by the locus prior to the DYT designation.
AD = autosomal dominant; AR = autosomal recessive; IP = incomplete penetrance; MRI = magnetic resonance imaging; XR = X-linked recessive.
Modified from Stacy 2001; Nemeth 2002.

may be impaired as a result of reduced reciprocal inhibition of H reflexes. The mechanism of impaired neuromuscular regulation is unknown, but may relate to cortical sensory processing. Electrophysiologic studies in a monkey model of focal dystonia have revealed the existence of single cells in hand regions of area 3b, with enlarged receptive fields extending to more than 1 digit, possibly causing abnormal processing of simultaneous sensory inputs. Functional magnetic resonance imaging (MRI) has been used to study abnormal processing of simultaneous sensory information in writer's cramp. Activation patterns for individual finger stimulation in controls demonstrated a 12% error, while patients with writer's cramp demonstrated a 30% error. In another functional MRI study, 8 patients with writer's cramp and 12 age-matched control subjects

TABLE 4.2 **Differential Diagnosis of Dystonia**

I. **Idiopathic (Primary) Dystonia**
  A. Sporadic (idiopathic torsion dystonia [ITD])
  B. Inherited (hereditary torsion dystonia)
    1. Autosomal-dominant ITD (DYT1)
    2. Autosomal-recessive tyrosine hydroxylase deficiency
II. **Secondary Dystonia**
  A. Dystonia-plus syndromes
    1. Myoclonic dystonia (not DYT1 gene)
    2. Dopa-responsive dystonia (guanosine triphosphate cyclohydrolase I; 14Q22.1-q22.2 gene defect)
    3. Rapid-onset dystonia—parkinsonism
    4. Early-onset parkinsonism with dystonia
    5. Paroxysmal dystonia—choreoathetosis
  B. Associated with neurodegenerative disorders
    1. Sporadic
      a. Parkinson's disease
      b. Progressive supranuclear palsy
      c. Multiple system atrophy
      d. Cortico-basal ganglionic degeneration
      e. Multiple sclerosis
      f. Central pontine myelinolysis
    2. Inherited
      a. Wilson's disease
      b. Huntington's disease
      c. Juvenile parkinsonism-dystonia
      d. Progressive pallidal degeneration
      e. Hallervorden-Spatz disease
      f. Hypoprebetalipoproteinemia, acanthocytosis, retinitis pigmentosa, and pallidal degeneration (HARP syndrome)
      g. Joseph's disease
      h. Ataxia telangiectasia
      i. Neuroacanthocytosis
      j. Rett's syndrome (?)
      k. Intraneuronal inclusion disease
      l. Infantile bilateral striatal necrosis
      m. Familial basal ganglia calcifications
      n. Spinocerebellar degeneration
      o. Olivopontocerebellar atrophy
      p. Hereditary spastic paraplegia with dystonia
      q. X-linked dystonia parkinsonism or Lubag (pericentromeric) deletion of 18q
  C. Associated with metabolic disorders
    1. Amino acid disorders
      a. Glutamic acidemia
      b. Methylmalonic acidemia
      c. Homocystenuria
      d. Hartnup's disease
      e. Tyrosinosis
    2. Lipid disorders
      a. Metachromatic leukodystrophy
      b. Ceroid lipofuscinosis
      c. Dystonic lipidosis ("sea-blue" histiocytosis)
      d. Gangliosidoses (GM1, GM2 variants)
      e. Hexosaminidase A and B deficiency
    3. Miscellaneous metabolic disorders
      a. Wilson's disease
      b. Mitochondrial encephalopathies (Leigh's disease, Leber's disease)
      c. Lesch-Nyhan syndrome
      d. Triosephosphate isomerase deficiency
      e. Vitamin E deficiency
      f. Biopterin deficiency
  D. Due to a known specific cause
    1. Perinatal cerebral injury and kernicterus (athetoid cerebral palsy, delayed-onset dystonia)
    2. Infection (viral encephalitis, encephalitis lethargica, Reye's syndrome, subacute sclerosing panencephalitis, Jakob-Creutzfeld disease, acquired immunodeficiency syndrome [AIDS])
    3. Other (tuberculosis, syphilis, acute infectious torticollis)
    4. Paraneoplastic brainstem encephalitis
    5. Cerebral vascular and ischemic injury
    6. Brain tumor
    7. Arteriovenous malformation
    8. Head trauma and brain surgery
    9. Peripheral trauma
    10. Toxins (Mn, CO, CS_2, methanol, disulfiram, wasp sting)
    11. Drugs (levodopa, bromocriptine, antipsychotic agents, metoclopramide, fenfluramine, flecainide, ergot agents, anticonvulsant agents, certain calcium channel–blocking agents)
III. **Other Hyperkinetic Syndromes Associated with Dystonia**
  A. Tic disorders with dystonic tics
  B. Paroxysmal dyskinesias
    1. Paroxysmal kinesigenic choreoathetosis
    2. Paroxysmal dystonic choreoathetosis
    3. Intermediate paroxysmal dyskinesia
    4. Benign infantile dyskinesia
IV. **Psychogenic**
V. **Pseudodystonia**
  A. Atlanto-axial subluxation
  B. Syringomyelia
  C. Arnold-Chiari malformation
  D. Trochlear nerve palsy
  E. Vestibular torticollis
  F. Posterior fossa mass
  G. Soft tissue neck mass
  H. Congenital postural torticollis
  I. Congenital Klippel-Feil syndrome
  J. Isaac's syndrome
  K. Sandiffer's syndrome
  L. Satoyoshi syndrome
  M. Stiff-person syndrome

Stacy 1999.

were given relaxation and contraction motor tasks involving the wrist. Activated volumes in the left sensorimotor cortex and the supplementary motor area were significantly reduced in patients for both muscle relaxation and contraction tasks when compared with controls.

While impairment of coordinated agonist–antagonist motor activity—perhaps secondary to reduced H-reflex inhibition—has been described, the mechanism for this physiologic change has not been elucidated. Both animal and human studies suggest that task-specific dystonia is associated with impaired cortical inhibition. These cortical changes likely result from striatal dysfunction. Altered thalamic activity has been proposed to play a role in the gaiting of cortical activity in dystonia. In this model, the patient at rest exhibits decreased thalamic activity to the cortex, while with movement, this activity is markedly increased. These thalamocortical circuit changes lead to alterations in spinal and brainstem reflexes and corticostriatal activity that may be attenuated by reduction in pallidal output. A recent study comparing 7 patients diagnosed with task-specific dystonia with 17 normal control subjects using 2-dimensional J-resolved magnetic resonance spectroscopy demonstrated that brain γ-aminobutyric acid (GABA) levels are decreased in the sensorimotor cortex and lentiform nuclei contralateral to the affected hand of the focal dystonia patients compared with the normal controls.

Another study of subjects with generalized dystonia undergoing muscle stretch reflex testing showed a significant reduction in the extent of the inhibitory phase after tendon-related excitation compared with a control group. It was suggested that electromyogram (EMG) suppression after tendon stimulation in the generalized dystonia population may be a result of dysfunction of presynaptic inhibitory mechanisms in the spinal cord, involving groups I and III afferents.

DIAGNOSTIC APPROACH

The diagnosis of primary dystonia should be considered in any patient with an abnormal posture. Information concerning age at onset, initial and subsequent areas of involvement, course and progression, tremor or other movement disorders, possible birth injury, developmental milestones, and exposure to neuroleptic medications, as well as a family history of dystonia, parkinsonism, or other movement disorders, should be reviewed. Since phenotypic expression of idiopathic torsion dystonia (ITD) is highly varied in this population, extreme care should be taken in recording family data with particular attention to consanguinity or Jewish ancestry. Evidence of other conditions known to produce dystonia but associated with other neurologic dysfunctions (e.g., cognitive, pyramidal, sensory, or cerebellar deficits) should also be considered. Ceruloplasmin should be obtained in all patients under the age of 50. Blood sample for genetic assessment, storage diseases, and metabolic disorders should be evaluated individually. Imaging of the brain (MRI or computed tomography scan) may be indicated in children and in adult-onset patients with a short history of limb dystonia.

MANAGEMENT

The majority of patients with writer's cramp may not present for medical care, and therefore not require any treatment. The use of writing aids has been advocated for patients with mild writing difficulty. A recent report of 5 patients with writer's cramp demonstrated improvement in writing ability with an applied hand orthosis. Another series of 11 professional musicians with task-specific finger dystonia underwent splint immobilization of the nonaffected digits for a period of 8 days. During this time, the subjects underwent daily supervised exercises with the dystonic finger for 30 to 60 minutes. After 1 year, benefit was seen in guitarists and pianists, but not in woodwind instrumentalists. Behavioral therapy or psychotherapy has not been effective.

Side effects of drug therapy for limb dystonia are often unacceptable to patients with task-specific dystonia—perhaps because symptoms are only present during specific activities. In subjects with more prominent or persistent involvement, oral medications may be appropriate. Anticholinergic drugs are effective in some, but the results are variable and are often associated with side effects such as blurred vision and drowsiness. In some patients with a component of tremor, β-blocking agents may be useful. Baclofen or tizanidine are commonly used in treating symptoms of dystonia, and may be most appropriate in patients with a history of hypoxic or traumatic brain injury. Benzodiazepines, particularly if patients report sleep difficulty, are also useful. In a series of 190 patients, approximately 1/3 experienced some benefit from medical therapy, which included anticholinergics, benzodiazepines, clonazepam, and diazepam. Because activation of globus pallidus internus (GPi) presynaptic cannabinoid receptors reduce GABA reuptake, and perhaps from patient anecdotal observation, it has been suggested that marijuana may reduce symptoms of dystonia. However, a double-blind, randomized, placebo-controlled, crossover study using the synthetic cannabinoid receptor agonist nabilone in patients with generalized and segmental primary dystonia showed no significant reduction in symptoms.

Botulinum toxin injections are highly effective in the treatment of limb dystonia. Injection strategy is determined by a combination of functional observation, muscle palpation, and electrophysiologic assessment. While muscle identification methods vary by clinician, functional assessment by observing the dystonic posture with the patient demonstrating the maximum change in posture is the most accurate identifier of muscles involved. However, increasing data suggest EMG guidance is useful in confirming toxin distribution to targeted muscles. A recent retrospective analysis of 235 patients receiving a total of 2,616 injections with botulinum toxin type A found continued benefit at 5 years. Interestingly, benefit was sustained in 100% of the lower limb–affected subjects, but only in 56% of the writer's cramp population. In this large series, 16.6% of patients developed resistance over the course of 10 years' follow-up. Adverse effects developed in 27% of patients at any single time, occurring over 4.5% of injection sessions, but were significantly lower in the limb dystonia groups. Currently, two botulinum serotypes (type A and type B) are available for commercial usage.

Perineural injection with 3% phenol has been used for 20 years in the management of spasticity in children, and may occasionally be considered in patients with spastic dystonia of a limb. This intervention requires considerable time, and the best results are seen with careful management of patient expectations and identification of potential response with injection of lidocaine prior to injection of phenol. Duration of benefit for spasticity ranges from 1 month to more than 2 years, and injection in the upper extremities generally shows greater benefit than in lower extremity procedures. Side effects include chronic dysesthesia and permanent nerve palsy. Motor point stimulation is useful for localization, and, although mixed motor and sensory nerves may be injected, injection of pure motor nerves (such as the musculocutaneous nerve) is associated with less pain.

Benefit from continuous and bolus intrathecal baclofen infusion was reported in a large group of subjects ranging in age from 3 to 42 years. All participants were diagnosed with generalized dystonia refractory to oral medications. In this series, improvement with bolus injections was reported in 80 of 86 subjects, and 77 participants underwent subsequent intrathecal catheter implantation. Of these subjects, 72 demonstrated benefit for a median follow-up period of up to 29 months. However, surgical complications, such as cerebrospinal fluid leaks, infections, and catheter problems, occurred in 29 subjects. Interestingly, a better response was noted when the catheter was placed above T-4, compared with the benefit seen with placement below T-6.

Functional stereotactic surgery should be considered in patients with disabling limb dystonia refractory to medical or botulinum toxin treatment. While most often this therapy is considered in patients with generalized or posttraumatic dystonia, in a series of 190 patients, surgery was successful in 27 of 29 cases. However, in 12 cases, results were transient. The success of ablation versus deep brain stimulation has not been compared, and the most appropriate target for surgical treatment (thalamic or pallidal) has not been determined. In a small series of 5 patients with generalized dystonia undergoing bilateral GPi pallidotomies, 4 patients with idiopathic dystonia showed a progressive improvement up to 3 months; the fifth patient, who had posttraumatic dystonia, did not benefit beyond this time.

Two cases of medically refractory, generalized dystonia treated by chronic high-frequency stimulation of the bilateral GPi have been reported. Greater than 80% reduction in the Burke-Fahn-Marsden Dystonia Movement Rating Scale was seen at 6 months, and continued for 24 months.

COST-EFFECTIVE TREATMENT OPTIONS FOR GENERALIZED DYSTONIA

In a treatment setting limited by financial concerns, the potential or confirmatory blood or imaging studies is likely unavailable. In this arena, evaluation and treatment of generalized dystonia relies heavily on careful history and physical examination. Since phenotypic expression of ITD is highly varied in this population, extreme care should be taken in recording family data with particular attention to consanguinity or Jewish ancestry. Given that an early onset of symptoms is predictive of ITD, this information is important for families to assist in planning for longer-term medical and caregiver support. Initial area(s) of involvement and pattern and rate of spread to other areas in an affected child also will assist parents and families in determining long-term care issues.

Historical issues not typically associated with idiopathic generalized dystonia include the presence of tremor or other movement disorders, possible birth injury, developmental milestones, and exposure to neuroleptic medications, as well as a family history of dystonia, parkinsonism, or other movement disorders. Identification of any of these risk factors may mean major differences in symptom progression, and may require different types of interventions. Evidence of other conditions known to produce dystonia but associated with other neurologic dysfunctions (e.g., cognitive, pyramidal, sensory, or cerebellar deficits) should also be considered.

Treatment of generalized dystonia in a setting in which the use of botulinum toxin, a baclofen pump, or surgical intervention are not options will rely heavily on assistive devices and oral medications. While physical and occupational therapy have not been demonstrated to alter the progression of ITD, daily range-of-motion sessions done by a caregiver will be helpful in reducing limb contracture. In some settings, the use of upper and lower limb bracing may also improve function and patient independence, but careful attention must be focused on the development of skin breakdown. Perhaps most importantly, investment in a durable, and perhaps individually designed, wheelchair is needed. Careful attention must be paid to the age of the patient, and deferring major expenditures for a long-term wheelchair is not recommended until the child has reached a growth plateau. Concurrent medical therapy most often includes treatment with levodopa, trihexyphenidyl, baclofen, or tizanidine, or a benzoidiazepine, as discussed earlier in this chapter.

COST-EFFECTIVE TREATMENT OPTIONS FOR LIMB DYSTONIA

A cost-effective approach for limb dystonia, regardless of whether it is in a generalized or focal setting, relies heavily on therapy and bracing. Medications such as those discussed above may also be helpful, but often sleepiness, cognitive disturbances, or other side effects preclude their utility—especially in the setting of a task-specific dystonia such as writer's cramp. However, any patient presenting with intermittent cramping of a limb, whether resting tremor is present or not, should receive a 1- to 2-month trial of levodopa (300 mg/day) to rule out the potential of Parkinson's disease of dopa-responsive dystonia. Although controlled trials of therapy are limited, some success has been reported in musicians with task-specific hand dystonia. The approach of splinting the nonaffected fingers while exercising the affected fingers daily for 8 days has shown modest benefit, and may allow for some return of nondystonia limb function to persist for as long as 1 year. Bracing in the lower limb should be considered to make every attempt to preserve ambulation, and may also require a cane or wheeled walker. Finally and in only a small percentage of patients, injection of phenol as a 3% solution may improve range of motion in some limbs. It should be emphasized that this approach is most useful to assist in hygiene control, and to prevent skin breakdown. Injections are better tolerated when motor nerves (e.g., musculocutaneous) rather than mixed nerves are treated.

CONCLUSIONS

The recognition and treatment of generalized and limb dystonia is often an extremely rewarding aspect of neurologic practice. In many instances, patients and families have not been given a clear diagnosis of an organic disorder, and thus diagnosis alone often improves patient well being. With careful workup, patients may benefit from medications or splint intervention; each patient should be given ample opportunity to respond to more than one medication. If botulinum toxin is available, this agent will often produce a gratifying response that will last for many years. However, in the generalized dystonia population, stereotactic neurosurgery may be the only real treatment option. In these situations, GPi ablation or stimulation has been found to be safe, but long-term efficacy data are not yet available.

ADDITIONAL READING

Chuang C, Fahn S, Frucht SJ. The natural history and treatment of acquired hemidystonia: report of 33 cases and review of the literature. *J Neurol Neurosurg Psychiatry* 2002;72:59–67.

Cohen LG, Hallett M, Sudarsky L. A single family with writer's cramp, essential tremor, and primary writing tremor. *Mov Disord* 1987;2:109–116.

Easton JK, Ozel T, Halpern D. Intramuscular neurolysis for spasticity in children. *Arch Phys Med Rehabil* 1979;60:155–158.

Jankovic J, Fahn S. Dystonic disorders. In: Jankovic J, Tolosa E, (eds.) *Parkinson's Disease and Movement Disorders*. 3rd ed. Baltimore: Williams & Wilkins; 1998.

Jankovic J. Post-traumatic movement disorders: central and peripheral mechanisms. *Neurology* 1994;44:2006–2014.

Karp BI, Cole RA, Cohen LG, Grill S, Lou JS, Hallett M. Long-term botulinum toxin treatment of focal hand dystonia. *Neurology* 1994;44(1):70–76.

Molloy FM, Shill HA, Kaelin-Lang A, Karp BI. Accuracy of muscle localization without EMG: implications for treatment of limb dystonia. *Neurology* 2002;58:805–807.

Nemeth AH. The genetics of primary dystonias and related disorders. *Brain* 2002;125:695–721.

Tarsy D. Comparison of acute- and delayed-onset posttraumatic cervical dystonia. *Mov Disord* 1998;13:481–485.

Tsui JKC, Bhatt M, Calne S, Calne DB. Botulinum toxin in the treatment of writer's cramp: a double-blind study. *Neurology* 1993;43:183–185.

Vitek JL. Pathophysiology of dystonia: a neuronal model. *Mov Disord* 2002;17(suppl 3):S49–S62.

Zafonte RD, Munin MC. Phenol and alcohol blocks for the treatment of spasticity. *Phys Med Rehabil Clin N Am* 2001;12:817–832.

CHAPTER 5

MEDICAL AND SURGICAL TREATMENT OF DYSTONIA

M. Fiorella Contarino, MD and Alberto Albanese, MD

INTRODUCTION

Dystonia has long remained a disorder with no effective treatments. Historically, it has been observed that some patients benefited from high doses of anticholinergic treatment and some from levodopa. We know now that the latter patients are affected by dopa-responsive dystonia (DRD). Most progress has been made in the late 1980s through the introduction of botulinum toxin (BoNT) for the treatment of focal or segmental dystonia. A number of therapeutic strategies are currently available to alleviate the symptoms of cervical dystonia. Oral medications include anticholinergic agents, dopamine receptor antagonists, and γ-aminobutyric acid (GABA)-mimetic agents. For the most part, the efficacy of these drugs is very limited, although roughly 40% of patients derive some symptomatic relief from anticholinergic agents. BoNTs have a high rate of efficacy combined with a low incidence of side effects and are considered the first choice in therapy for several forms of focal dystonia. Pharmacologic management of dystonia with oral agents or BoNT is symptomatic, not curative. In patients who fail to respond to medical therapy, surgical approaches may be appropriate. Surgical options include selective peripheral denervation, bilateral pallidotomy, or globus pallidum deep brain stimulation.

The appropriate treatment choice depends on the exact diagnosis, because dystonia can be one of the symptoms of neurodegenerative diseases or a primary disorder (see Chapter 1, "Diagnosis, Classification, and Pathophysiology of Dystonia"). In a small, but sizable, percentage of dystonia patients, specific etiologic treatment can cure dystonia (e.g., DRD, Wilson's disease, psychogenic dystonia, tardive dystonia, etc.), but in the remaining majority, dystonia can be treated only symptomatically. A problem with the evaluation of treatments for dystonia is the paucity of randomized controlled studies, which reflects in part the high variability of the phenomenology and also the late development of validated rating scales. Rating scales have so far been validated only for cranial and cervical dystonia.

As a general rule, five basic treatment options are available: (1) BoNT injection, (2) oral and intrathecal pharmacotherapy, (3) physical therapies, (4) surgical therapy, and (5) supportive/social treatment (Table 5.1). Combination therapies may be appropriate. For those who cannot be treated effectively with BoNT, pharmacotherapy can be tried. Pharmacotherapy may also alleviate symptoms that remain after BoNT therapy. Physical therapies are recommended for most patients receiving BoNT to extend the benefits. BoNT may change movement patterns; thus, physical therapies may help patients relearn normal postures and functional control. Surgical options should be reserved for patients refractory to all conservative treatment approaches (Figure 5.1).

TREATMENTS FOR SPECIFIC FORMS OF DYSTONIA

Specific treatments, directed toward the underlying biochemical defects, are available for some forms of dystonia.

Dopa-Responsive Dystonia

DRD is associated with a deficiency of guanosine-5'-triphosphate (GTP) cyclohydrolase 1 or tyrosine hydroxylase activity in nigrostriatal terminals. Levodopa is the most appropriate treatment to restore the lack of dopamine. Most patients improve with low doses (<500 mg/day) of levodopa combined with a peripheral decarboxylase inhibitor. Rarely, higher dosages are required. Levodopa provides symptomatic relief that compensates for the causative metabolic defect and must be continued for life. Unlike Parkinson's disease, levodopa-related side effects—such as nausea, constipation, orthostatic hypotension, confusion, and hallucinations—are uncommon in DRD patients, and resolve with dose reduction. Fluctuations or dyskinesias similar to those occurring in Parkinson's disease are also observed in DRD, particularly when high doses of levodopa are prescribed, and usually resolve with dose reduction. Genetic testing for DRD allows for identification of patients who carry the

TABLE 5.1 Available Treatments for Dystonia and Their Indications

Treatment	Generalized and segmental	Focal
Botulinum toxin	Indicated if focal symptoms are prevalent and are a significant cause of disability or pain	First-choice indication in most forms
Pharmacotherapy	Oral medications	Oral medications, as indicated for generalized and segmental dystonia
	• Levodopa/carbidopa (to diagnose and treat DRD), anticholinergics, baclofen, benzodiazepines, dopamine depletors (tetrabenazine), "triple therapy"	
	Intrathecal baclofen	
Surgery	CNS surgery	Peripheral surgery
	• Deep brain stimulation, pallidotomy, thalamotomy	• Rarely indicated
		Central surgery
		• Pallidal DBS is to be evaluated in large series
Physical and supportive	Indicated in most cases	Indicated in most cases

CNS=central nervous system; DBS=deep brain stimulation; DRD=dopa-responsive dystonia.

genetic defect, although a number of patients may escape genetic diagnosis due to sporadic presentation or to genetic heterogeneity. For this reason, a trial of levodopa is warranted in all patients with childhood- or adolescent-onset dystonia. Dopamine agonists, such as bromocriptine, apomorphine, and lisuride have also proven efficacious in DRD.

Wilson's Disease

Pharmacologic treatment of Wilson's disease blocks the buildup of copper or reverses its toxic effects on the brain and other organs. This can be obtained in a number of ways: (1) reduction of copper absorption, (2) induction of synthesis of endogenous cellular proteins such as metallothioneine (which is capable of sequestering copper in a nontoxic manner within cells), (3) promotion of the excretion of copper, or (4) combination of >1 approach. Pharmacologic agents that remove copper, such as D-penicillamine, trientine, and tetrathiomolibdate, are chelating agents. Zinc stimulates metallothioneine in enterocytes and blocks absorption of copper from food. Trientine is a good candidate for initial treatment. Combination therapy (chelating and zinc) may be useful in treating some symptomatic patients.

SYMPTOMATIC TREATMENTS OF DYSTONIAS

Oral Treatments

Anticholinergic Agents

Anticholinergic agents are thought to act on striatal cholinergic interneurons to improve dystonia. High doses are required and the clinical efficacy is limited by side effects. In addition, their symptomatic effects may not be stable over time. The main indication for the use of anticholinergic drugs is generalized dystonia; the best-studied agent is trihexyphenidyl. Treatment with this drug produces an appreciable benefit in 40% to 50% of patients. Low doses (1 mg/day) are slowly increased until an effective regimen is reached over several months. Usually, daily doses of 80 to 120 mg (or up to 180 mg in children) are used. Clinical benefit is reached only after several weeks. Trihexyphenidyl is more effective in children, who tolerate higher doses than adults. The best results are obtained if the treatment is introduced within 5 years of onset.

Side effects of anticholinergic drugs are central and peripheral. Central effects include confusion, memory impairment, hallucinations, restlessness, insomnia, nightmares, and sedation. Peripheral side effects (such as dry mouth, blurred vision, exacerbation of acute angle glaucoma, urinary retention, and constipation) may be controlled by peripheral cholinergic drugs, such as pyridostigmine or pilocarpine. Side effects

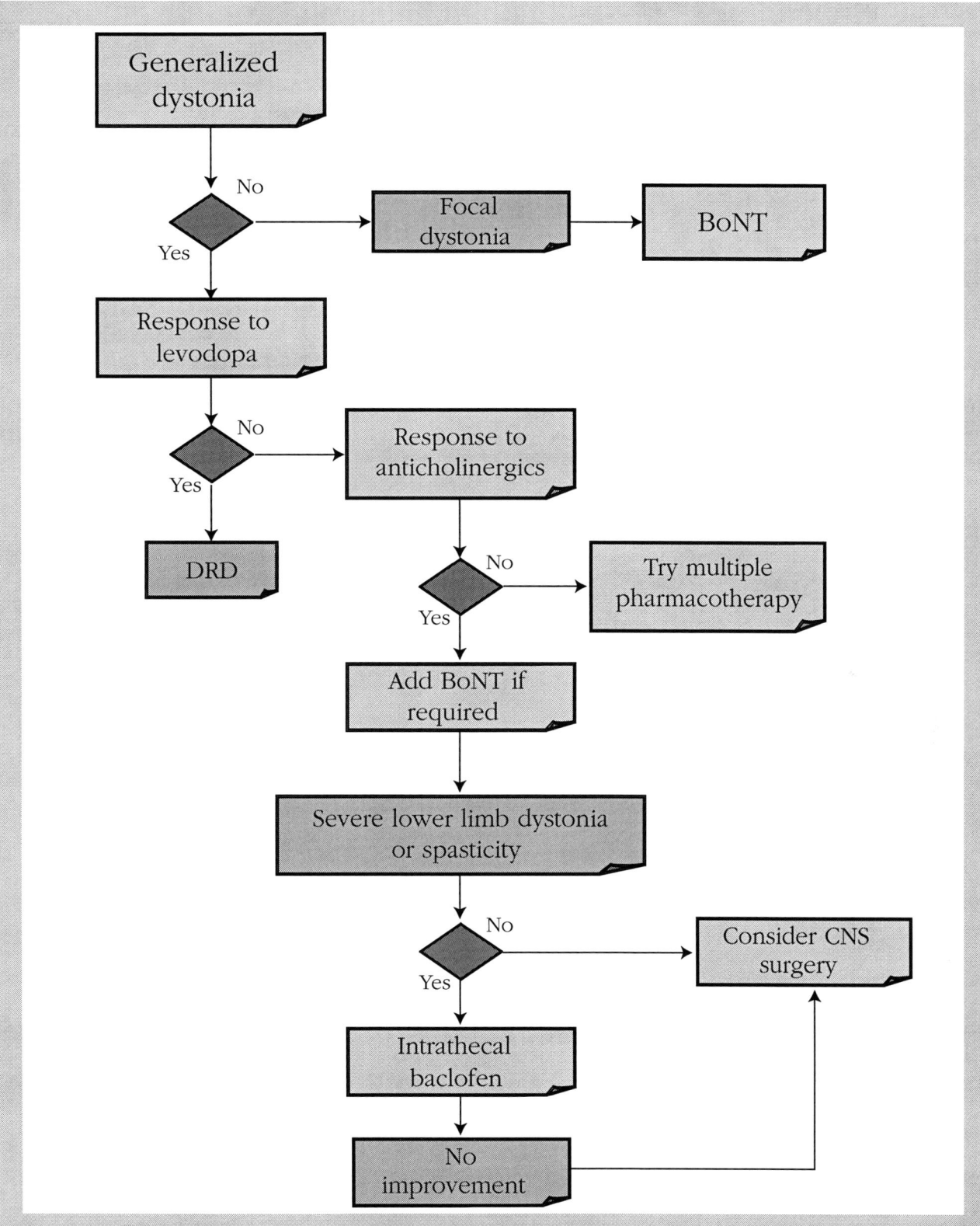

FIGURE 5.1 Flow chart of clinical decisions for the treatment of generalized dystonia. BoNT=botulinum toxin; CNS=central nervous system; DRD=dopa-responsive dystonia.

(especially central ones) are more frequent in the elderly and are usually dose related. Abrupt withdrawal of anticholinergic drugs may induce cholinergic symptoms (such as nausea, diarrhea, and bradycardia) or exacerbation of dystonia. In addition to trihexyphenidyl, the following anticholinergic agents have occasionally provided benefit to dystonia: benztropine, ethopropazine, biperiden, atropine, procyclidine, orphenadrine, and scopolamine (also through transdermal delivery).

Neuroleptic Drugs

Classic neuroleptics have been employed to treat severe dystonia. Their use is still controversial, because some studies have reported efficacy (improvement of 11%–30%), while others have not. However, side effects of classic neuroleptics (such as sedation, apathy, nausea, orthostatic hypotension, insomnia, akathisia, and confusion) and the risk of producing tardive dyskinesias now greatly limit their usage.

Tetrabenazine is a presynaptic monoamine-depleting drug that also blocks postsynaptic dopamine receptors. It can be used alone or in association with other antidystonic drugs. Tetrabenazine is particularly efficacious in about 85% of patients with drug-induced dystonia and in >70% of patients with primary dystonia. Treatment is started at low doses (12.5 mg q.i.d. or b.i.d.) and increased on a monthly schedule until efficacious or side effects occur. The optimal dose ranges from 25 to 400 mg/day. Tardive side effects are much more rare than following the administration of classic neuroleptics, but transient acute dystonic reactions have also been reported with tetrabenazine. Side effects include, by decreasing incidence: drowsiness or fatigue (36.5% of cases), parkinsonian features (28.5%), depression (15.0%), insomnia (11.0%), akathisia (9.5%), acute dystonic reaction (2.8%), tremor (2.5%), and memory impairment or confusion (2.3%). Dysphoria has occasionally been described. Depression can be severe and life threatening if not recognized and prevented by a dose reduction. The efficacy of tetrabenazine is usually observed in <2 weeks. Little evidence has been collected on the use of reserpine, a dopamine-depleting agent, which may have an indication for tardive dystonia. A particular type of neuroleptic treatment, which has been used mainly during the past decade, is so-called "triple therapy," combining tetrabenazine, one classic neuroleptic, and an anticholinergic drug.

Atypical neuroleptics, such as clozapine, olanzapine, or risperidone have been used anecdotally to treat tardive dystonia, especially in patients who require neuroleptic treatment for psychosis. Their use in primary dystonia is poorly documented.

Benzodiazepines

Benzodiazepines have been used in dystonia for >3 decades, alone or in association with anticholinergic drugs. No controlled study has documented their efficacy under oral administration. Clonazepam and diazepam are the most often used drugs. High doses are required to achieve benefit, and a gradual increase in dose is often necessary to prevent side effects. Sedation and ataxia are the limiting side effects in most patients. Withdrawal symptoms, including worsening of dystonia, occur if the doses are lowered suddenly. Depression, confusion, and dependence may occur. Successful treatment has been reported on dystonia associated with corticobasal degeneration or Parkinson's disease (9%), paroxysmal dystonic head tremor, tardive dystonia, blepharospasm, and myoclonic dystonia.

Baclofen

There have been no controlled studies of the use of oral baclofen in dystonia. Retrospective studies found it effective at high doses (92 mg, range 40–180 mg) in 29% of children with generalized dystonia. Adults with dystonia are less likely to benefit from oral baclofen, and improvement is less dramatic when it occurs. Baclofen is usually initiated at a dose of 10 mg b.i.d. or t.i.d. The dose may be increased slowly to a total of 120 mg (t.i.d. or q.i.d.), unless side effects are observed. Frequently reported side effects include nausea, sedation, and muscle weakness. Lethargy, dizziness, dysphoria, dry mouth, and urinary urgency or hesitation may also occur, while confusion, hallucinations, and paranoia have been reported rarely. Once initiated, the drug should be discontinued slowly, because abrupt cessation may cause serious symptoms such as psychosis or seizures or increase in dystonia.

Baclofen can be delivered intrathecally into the lumbar subarachnoid space by using an implantable and refillable device. Efficacy must be tested before the implant by the acute administration of incremental bolus infusions (usually from 50 to 100 µg). Some patients may respond to higher doses, but side effects of high-dose regimens included central nervous system depression, hypotension, or respiratory arrest. Common side effects reported in the acute challenge include paresthesias, limb weakness, dizziness, and headache. Adverse reactions may be temporarily reversed by physostigmine. Following the acute challenge, continuous delivery usually is set for 24 hours; the effective trial dose is increased by 10% to 30%, without exceeding a total dose of 800 µg/day. However, in selected patients, doses up to 1500 µg/day have been used for delivery. The best placement for the catheter is at T4 rather than at T6 or at a lower level of the spinal cord.

It has been reported that patients without improvement (or with equivocal results) after repeated bolus injections may still benefit from a continuous delivery of baclofen. On the other hand, approximately 40% of patients whose symptoms ameliorated during the acute test may have poor long-term benefit.

Intrathecal baclofen is more effective in patients with trunk and lower limb dystonia, but it is also efficacious on coexisting spasticity. In fact, lower doses of baclofen are generally required to improve spasticity than dystonia, when they occur in combination. This also explains why baclofen is more effective on secondary than on primary dystonia. Side effects of long-term infusion include tolerance (probably due to a down-regulation of spinal GABA-B receptors), over- or underdelivery (due to malfunction or inappropriate programming of the system), local infection, and catheter malfunction. Complications related to the surgical procedure are not uncommon (up to 38%) and include cerebrospinal fluid leakage, infections, or catheter-related problems.

The initial capital outlay for the drug-infusion system, including the cost of the device, the procedure, and the hospital stay is estimated at approximately € 18,000 to € 22,000, with an initial cost of about € 350 for filling the pump with baclofen. Moreover, the pump needs to be refilled periodically. Although this is not an irrelevant cost, the system is valuated to be quite cost effective.

Other Medical Treatments

Many other drugs have been tested in patients with dystonia, before the advent of BoNT, but the experimentation of new agents has diminished markedly in recent years.

Carbamazepine and other anticonvulsants, such as phenytoin, gabapentin and valproic acid, have an indication for paroxysmal dyskinesias such as paroxysmal kinesigenic choreoathetosis or nocturnal paroxysmal dystonia.

Cannabinoids have been considered an indication for dystonia because stimulation of cannabinoid receptors has been shown to reduce overactivity in the globus pallidum internum (GPi) and thereby improve dystonia. However, the synthetic cannabinoid agonist nabilone produced no effect on dystonia.

Several other drugs, acting via different mechanisms (such as riluzole, tizanidine, methylprednisolone, mexiletine, dantrolene, amphetamine, cyproheptidine, 5-hydroxytryptophan, calcitonin, lithium, diphenhydramine, and acetazolamide) have been anecdotally tried on dystonia patients without any valuable result.

BoNT

BoNT has been used to treat dystonia since 1984 and has become a first-line treatment for many focal forms. Segmental and generalized dystonias are approached as a collection of focal treatments. There are 7 serologically distinct BoNTs (named from A to G). BoNT A and B are commercially available for clinical use. They all produce a local chemodenervation by inhibiting the release of acetylcholine from neuromuscular synapses. Each BoNT serotype acts on 1 of the proteins that allow synaptic vesicles (containing acetylcholine) to fuse with the presynaptic membrane and release their content in the synaptic cleft. The action of BoNT produces a flaccid paralysis of the injected muscle.

Commercial versions of BoNT include Botox® (Allergan, Irvine, CA) and Dysport® (Ipsen Slough, Berkshire, UK) both BoNT type A and Myobloc™ (Neurobloc™ in Europe, Solstice Neurosciences, San Diego, CA) is a BoNT type B (Figure 5.2). The clinical indications of these 3 toxins are similar, but differ from one country to another due to local differences in registration processes. The price of BoNT varies quite significantly among countries; in Europe, for example, hospital prices for 1 vial of Botox® (100 U) ranges from € 210 (in Austria and Switzerland) to € 396 (in Slovakia), whereas that of a vial of Dysport® (500 U) varies from € 243 (in Austria) to € 433 (in Italy) (quotations for the year 2002). In Australia, 1 Botox® vial (100 U) costs AUD$450 (about $247 US; quotations for the year 2001).

The 3 BoNT brands have different potencies, which are calculated using independent units (Table 5.2). The equivalence of units is not strict. It can be calculated that 1 U Botox® corresponds to approximately 3 to 5 U Dysport® and to approximately 40 to 50 U Myobloc™, depending on the injected site and on the indication. Other differences exist between the 2 BoNT type A brands, such as storage or diffusion in tissue; therefore, switching a patient from 1 BoNT type A brand to the other requires a trial-and-error approach. A similar complication holds true when changing from a BoNT A preparation to BoNT B. Side effects of the different toxins are comparable. Preliminary, unconfirmed evidence suggests that Dysport® diffuses more than Botox® and that Myobloc™ injections may be more painful than those of BoNT A preparations. It has been hypothesized that BoNT B may produce more parasympathetic systemic side effects. In addition to those mentioned, other BoNT serotypes have been used in the clinic, such as BoNT C and F, with preliminary results.

Following an intramuscular injection, the toxin diffuses in the surrounding tissue. The size of the diffusion

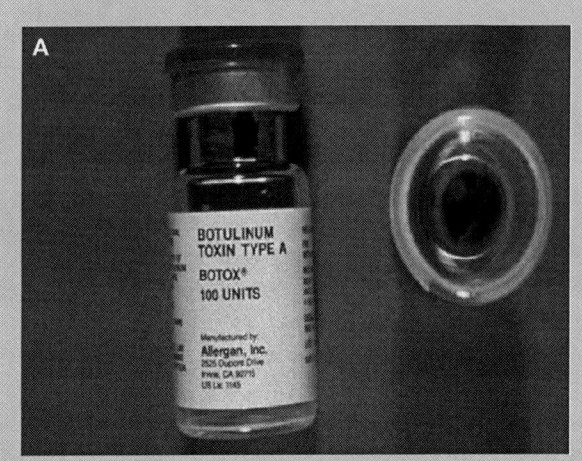

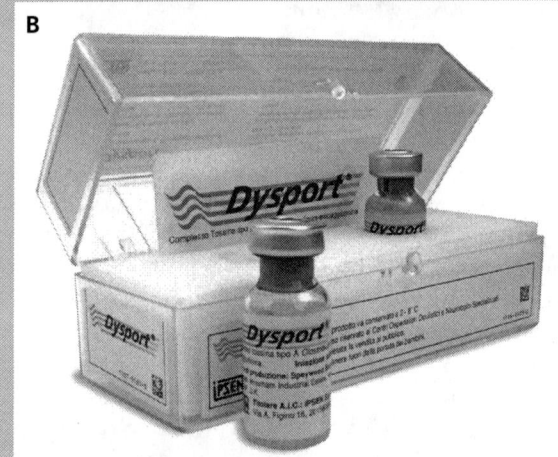

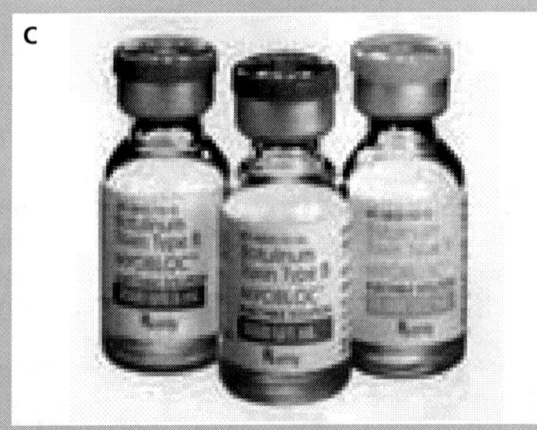

FIGURE 5.2 Botulinum toxin brands available for clinical use. (a) Botox® (Allergan, Irvine, CA); lyophilized type A toxin. (b) Dysport® (Ipsen Slough, Berkshire, UK); lyophilized type A toxin. (c) Myobloc™ (Solstice Neurosciences, San Diego, CA); liquid type B toxin.

area depends in part on the amount injected. For example, it is estimated that 1 U Botox® diffuses approximately 15 to 30 mm in diameter; 2.5 to 10 U Botox® diffuse 30 to 45 mm. It has been demonstrated by different techniques that small amounts of BoNT A or B can produce weakness in sites that are remote from the injected muscles. However, there is no evidence of generalized weakness in patients treated with the standard doses. The onset of action of BoNT A occurs within 3 to 5 days following an injection, and peaks at 2 to 4 weeks. The duration of benefit is 3 to 6 months. Whether the effects of BoNTs can be cumulative remains controversial. There is no evidence to suggest that BoNT treatment alters the natural history of dystonia, although long-term follow-up has shown prolonged symptomatic relief. Side effects usually resolve in a few weeks. Morphologic changes associated with long-term BoNT treatment consist of atrophy of neuromuscular plaques and sprouting of nerve terminals.

The limitations to the use of BoNT injections include: the inability to treat too many muscles because of concerns not to exceed the total recommended dose; difficulty in reaching muscles that are inaccessible or unsafe to inject (such as the prevertebral muscles, or the tongue); the occurrence of adverse effects. The manufacturers suggest not to exceed the following dose limits for the use of brand-name BoNTs. Allergan advises not to exceed a cumulative dose of 200 U Botox® in a 30-day period; Ipsen suggests a maximum dose of 1000 U Dysport® in each treatment session. Solstice Neurosciences sets the limit of a total maximum dose of 10,000 to 15,000 U Myobloc™ per treatment session and, in each injection site, a dose up to 2500 U Myobloc™ and a maximum volume not exceeding 0.5 mL.

Dystonia may be only partially corrected by BoNT; efficacy often is reduced after repeated treatments. From 6% to 14% of patients do not respond to BoNT at the first treatment (primary nonresponders); approximately 3% respond initially and then lose efficacy (secondary nonresponders). Primary or secondary resistance may be due to the production of neutralizing antibodies to the BoNT serotype used. There are 2 main reasons for a patient to develop secondary response loss: (1) inappropriate treatment (incorrect muscle choice or inappropriate dose), and (2) development of antibodies to the BoNT serotype used. The first reason is by far the most common. Inappropriate treatment may be caused by a too-rigid injection scheme, not taking into account the changing nature of muscle activation in dystonia. The experienced neurologist would modify the muscle selection and the doses injected to follow the changing pattern of dystonia.

TABLE 5.2   Manufactured Brands of Botulinum Toxins

Feature	Botox®	Dysport®	Myobloc™
Serotype	A	A	B
Specific activity	20 U/ng	40 U/ng	70–130 U/ng
Packaging	100 U/vial	500 U/vial	2500; 5000; 10,000 U/vial
Constituents and excipients	Human albumin; sodium chloride	Hemagglutinin; human albumin 20% solution; lactose	Hemagglutinin and nonhemagglutinin proteins; human albumin solution 0.05%; sodium chloride; sodium succinate (pH 5.6)
Preparation	Lyophilized	Lyophilized	Solution (5000 U/mL)
Storage of packaged product	-5°C	2–8°C	2–8°C
Storage once reconstituted	2–8°C for 4 h	2–8°C for 8 h	2–8°C for 4 h (if diluted)

Antibodies are produced in 5% to 10% of patients who receive injections in the cervical muscles or in other large muscles. Only 33% of secondary nonresponder patients have demonstrable circulating antibodies. The remaining 2/3 of secondary nonresponding patients are thought to have a cause different from antibody production for their secondary resistance. The incidence of antibody formation may be underestimated, because available tests are highly specific, but poorly sensitive. The occurrence of neutralizing antibodies can be indirectly demonstrated by lack of weakness after an appropriate BoNT injection in a specific muscle (e.g., the frontalis muscle). Predisposing factors to the production of antibodies include: a short interval between treatments (less than 3 months) and the use of high doses (>300 U Botox® per treatment session). Young age is also considered to be a predisposing factor. In patients with complete secondary resistance, it is inappropriate to increase BoNT dose; however, in patients with partial secondary failure, this approach might restore the previous efficacy of BoNT without inducing appreciable side effects. Patients who develop antibodies to BoNT A may benefit from injections of a distinct BoNT serotype (e.g., BoNT B).

As a general rule, side effects following BoNT treatment are related to excessive weakness produced in the injected or in nearby muscles. In addition, skin rushes or flulike symptoms have been reported. Contraindications to BoNT injections are a history of allergic reactions, pregnancy, muscle or local inflammation or an infection in the injection site. Other contraindications to be thoroughly evaluated are the coexistence of a neuromuscular disease (myasthenia gravis, Lambert-Eaton syndrome, polyradiculoneuritis, amyotrophic lateral sclerosis, etc.), or the concomitant administration of drugs interfering with neuromuscular transmission (such as aminoglycosides, antimicrobials, penicillamine, quinine, and calcium antagonists).

Blepharospasm

BoNT stands as the primary indication for blepharospasm; a significant improvement is reported in about 93% of patients (70% to 100%). The average duration of efficacy is approximately 12 weeks. The doses injected around each eye are usually divided into 4 to 5 points and range from 12.5 to 25 U Botox®, 100 to 125 U Dysport®, or 750 to 2500 U Myobloc™, but may be increased in individual cases. Unsatisfactory results occur in about 6% to 7% of patients. The injection technique can affect the outcome: injecting BoNT A in the pretarsal rather than in the orbital portion of the orbicularis oculi muscle may increase the success rate and decrease the incidence of side effects. Repeated BoNT treatments do not yield to loss of efficacy, as observed after an 11-year follow-up. Common side effects are ptosis (13.4 %), kheratitis (4.1%), epiphora (3.5%), dry eyes, diplopia, and lid edema. Less frequent complications include: facial weakness, lagophtalmos, ecchymosis, ectropion or entropion, or local pain. Side effects usually resolve in about 2 weeks.

Cervical Dystonia

The outcome of BoNT treatment is more variable in cervical dystonia than in blepharospasm, with a success rate approaching 70% (40%–90%; Table 5.3). Most

TABLE 5.3	Botulinum Toxin: Efficacy in Focal Dystonias
Indication	**Efficacy rate**
Blepharospasm	69%–100%
Cervical dystonia	70% (39%–90%)
Oromandibular closing dystonia	70%
Oromandibular opening dystonia	50%
Laryngeal adductory dystonia	Appox. 100%
Limbs dystonia and professional dystonia	Variable

patients report reduction of pain, but the outcome concerning the movement disorder itself is less predictable. The doses injected are divided into 2 to 3 points per muscle and are greatly variable according to presentation. The standard doses are up to 100 to 250 U Botox®, 500 to 1000 U Dysport®, or 5000 to 10,000 U Myobloc™. The latency of effects varies from 3 to 7 days in the majority of cases, and often peaks at 1 week. The duration of effects is variable between patients and within a single patient. On average, a complete effect lasts approximately about 12 weeks (ranging from 4 to 24 weeks). Doses vary between patients and depend on the clinical presentation, including the muscles involved, disease severity, and the use of concomitant medication. Electromyogram (EMG) guidance has proven useful in all cases that do not improve adequately following a treatment under visual guidance. Patients with a longer history of disease achieve less benefit than those in the early stages; there are several possible explanations for this observation, such as the occurrence of more complex muscle activation patterns with advanced disease or the development of structural abnormalities of tendons and muscles.

Side effects occur in approximately 20% to 30% of treatments, and can usually be managed. A potentially life-threatening side effect is dysphagia, which is usually caused by diffusion following injections placed in the sternocleidomastoid muscles; other common side effects include weakness of the cervical muscles or pain at injection sites. These usually resolve within 2 to 3 weeks.

The outcome following BoNT B treatment seems to be similar to that reported with BoNT A. However, no controlled trials directly comparing the 2 serotypes have been conducted to date.

Oromandibular Dystonia

For mouth-closing dystonia, the masseter muscles are injected bilaterally with approximately 30 U Botox® in each side. Improvement in mastication and speech is obtained in approximately 70% of patients. Early treatment can prevent tooth damage. In mouth-opening dystonia, the lateral pterygoid muscles or the digastric muscles can be injected (mean dose 20 U Botox®). The outcome rate is about 50%; side effects consist of dysphagia (approximately 20% of cases).

Laryngeal Dystonia

In adductor spasmodic dysphonia, the thyroarytenoid muscle is injected, usually under EMG guidance or, less frequently, by direct laryngoscopy. Clinical improvement lasts for approximately 3 to 6 months. Outcome rate is around 100%. Doses injected are in the range of 5 U Botox® or 30 to 40 U Dysport® on each side. Treatment is beneficial, despite different techniques used, in 75% to 95% of patients. Side effects include hypophonia and dysphagia.

Laryngeal abductor spasmodic dysphonia is more difficult to treat, because the muscle responsible for the spasmodic contractions is the cricoarytenoid muscle—the only abductor muscle of the larynx, whose excessive weakness may cause life-threatening laryngospasm. Treatment is usually performed under the direct surveillance of an ear, nose, and throat surgeon.

Occupational Cramps and Upper Limb Dystonia

Upper limb dystonia is not uncommon and often appears in the form of task-specific occupational dystonia. Motor control of the upper limb depends on a large variety of muscles, which must be injected individually with BoNT under EMG guidance. This treatment requires experience, and various combinations of injections have to be tried in some patients. The outcome is often unsatisfactory in professional performers (such as musicians), who require skilled control of upper limb movements. BoNT injections are placed in a variety of muscles, such as the carpal flexors, carpal extensors, pronators, supinator, triceps, biceps, brachialis, brachioradialis, finger flexors, or extensors.

BoNT treatment can be combined with splinting to improve outcome, particularly for torsional dystonic movements.

Lower Limb Dystonia

Foot dystonia, either primary (as in the case of generalized dystonia) or secondary (e.g., in Parkinson's disease), can be treated with BoNT to obtain pain relief and improvement of function.

Surgical Treatment

Peripheral Surgery

Peripheral surgical denervation has been used to treat blepharospasm, spasmodic dysphonia, and cervical dystonia. This technique implies cutting nerves or muscles. There are no controlled trials on peripheral surgery for dystonia, and available studies report a significant variability of assessments and procedures. For these reasons, and for the scantiness of follow-up data, the efficacy of these treatments has not been proved. Adequate results depend mainly on the training and experience of the surgeon and the careful selection of patients. Peripheral surgery should be reserved for patients who do not respond to more conservative treatments, such as medications, BoNT injections, or stereotactic interventions.

In patients with blepharospasm, peripheral facial neurectomy has been performed using alcohol injections, surgical sectioning, selective peripheral nerve avulsion, and percutaneous nerve thermolysis. All these procedures have been limited by the occurrence of permanent complications, such as paralytic ectropion, lagophtalmos, epiphora, upper lid dermatochalasis, lip paresis, dropping of the mouth, and loss of facial expression. Selective myectomy is obtained by removing one or more of the following muscles: upper orbicularis oculi, procerus, or corrugator supercilii. Complications include numbness of the forehead, chronic lymphedema of the periorbital region, exposure keratitis, ptosis or ectropion, and lid retraction.

In the treatment of dysphonia, section of the recurrent laryngeal nerve was initially reported to produce dramatic improvement, but long-term follow-up evaluations have later documented that only a minority of patients (approximately 36%) had persistent benefit, while 48% of patients were worse than before. Side effects were numerous.

Type I thyroplasty has been performed in selected patients with abductor laryngeal dystonia. This reversible procedure brings 1 arytenoid muscle closer to the midline.

Selective peripheral denervation (such as extradural section of nerve roots, or ramisectomy) has yielded variable results in patients with cervical dystonia. Patients with torticollis had better results than patients with laterocollis or retrocollis. Side effects include sensory deficits, weakness of the trapezius, dysphagia, occipital neuralgia, and dysesthesias. Ramisectomy has also been associated with a section of the spinal accessory nerve; this was based on the hypothesis that dystonia may originate from altered proprioception, caused by mechanical irritation of an anastomosis between the spinal accessory nerve and C1 or C2 dorsal roots. Bilateral anterior cervical rhizotomies combined with a selective section of the spinal accessory nerve (or an intradural section of nerve roots) have caused a high rate of permanent postoperative neck weakness.

Myotomies of posterior neck muscles consist of a partial section of the superior trapezius muscle, a section of the splenius capitis, and a section of the semispinalis. These procedures have been performed occasionally on patients with retrocollis.

Necrotizing drugs, such as the toxic agent doxorubicin, can also produce myectomy and denervation. This approach has little clinical application, due to severe local irritation. Rather, injection of phenol, which causes coagulation of peripheral nerves, is used in the management of spasticity and has been investigated as a potential treatment of cervical dystonia. The results have not been very encouraging because of unpredictable response and side effects (local pain, chronic dysesthesias, excessive motor weakness, and sensory loss). Epidural cervical cord stimulation has provided no benefit.

Surgical procedures may be beneficial in appropriately selected patients, but require long postoperative recovery periods and may cause excessive neck weakness. Selective peripheral denervation is the only such technique of wide usage in cervical dystonia.

Central Nervous System Surgery

Surgery for the treatment of hyperkinetic movement disorders (including dystonia) dates back to the beginning of the 20th century.

Ablative Surgery

Stereotactic lesions, developed in the 1950s, were also aimed at correcting dystonia. Pallidotomy, and later thalamotomy, were indicated for the treatment of dystonia in the early days. A benefit of up to 60% was reported for pallidotomy in generalized primary dystonia. This seemed to persist over the long term. Improvement after bilateral or unilateral posteroventral pallidotomy has also been reported in cases of tardive dystonia.

The historical target for thalamotomy was the ventrolateral thalamus, where pallidofugal fibers are relayed. It is unclear to what extent thalamotomy acts by altering pallidal outflow to the thalamus. This procedure has continued until recently, more commonly with unilateral lesions. A significant benefit on the contralateral dystonic limbs has been reported in a variable percentage of patients (30%–70%). By contrast, little effect has been observed on axial dystonia, and a decrease in efficacy has been reported at 36-month follow-up. Appreciable results have also been obtained in secondary dystonia with unilateral thalamotomy targeted on the anterior part of ventrolateral nucleus. An improvement has been observed in 62% of patients with cervical dystonia treated with bilateral thalamotomy. Complications and side effects occur in up to 20% of patients following thalamotomy, and are often persistent. These effects are more frequent after a bilateral procedure. In recent years, the indication of thalamotomy has been greatly reduced, because of the variability of results obtained and the high incidence of permanent side effects (particularly dysarthria).

Deep Brain Stimulation

Compared with creating lesions, deep brain stimulation (DBS) is a more conservative and manageable approach. Side effects are less frequent, and the procedure is reversible and can be adapted to individual clinical features. DBS, however, is a more expensive procedure, as it requires implanted material (leads, internal pulse generators, and connectors). The internal pulse generator needs to be replaced periodically, usually after 2 to 3 years of continuous use. No randomized controlled trials have been performed on stereotactic surgery—either ablation or stimulation.

Thalamic DBS (targeted to the Vim nucleus) has no proven efficacy in generalized dystonia. As for cervical dystonia, relief has been reported for pain and partially for dystonic movements. Pallidal DBS (targeted to the ventroposterolateral part of the internal pallidum, just above the optic tract) has produced encouraging results in patients with primary generalized dystonia. An improvement of up to 81.3% has been observed on clinical scales for dystonia, and, particularly, in a subgroup of patients with DYT1 dystonia who had a striking improvement of 90.3%. Other anecdotal reports have mentioned poor results on DYT1 cases.

The improvement in motor symptoms arises gradually, within hours or days. Additive improvement on dystonic postures has been reported after over 1 year of stimulation. Pallidal stimulation, but not thalamic stimulation, seems to be effective in secondary dystonia as well; however, the efficacy of pallidal DBS in focal and segmental forms remains more questionable. The available data are still insufficient to draw indications for DBS in secondary or focal dystonia cases (Figure 5.3). A different approach based on low-frequency stimulation of the subthalamic nucleus has recently been proposed, on the basis of a presumed excitatory effect.

According to manufacturer information, costs of a DBS device to hospitals in Europe for monolateral stimulation amount to approximately € 7,600 (approximately € 15,200 for bilateral stimulation; quotation for the year 2000). Considering the daily cost of a hospital stay (usually as long as 20 days) of approximately € 243, total costs for performing a bilateral DBS implant rise to approximately € 20,000 to € 25,000. In the United States, the cost of a bilateral DBS implant ranges on average from $50,000 to $60,000. This estimate varies depending on the length of hospital stay.

Physical and Supportive Treatments

Patient education, physical therapy, and supportive care are integral and critical elements of a comprehensive treatment scheme. No controlled studies have been performed to support the efficacy of physical therapy. The best therapeutic results are obtained when systemic medication, BoNT injections, and physiotherapy are combined.

It is worth remembering that reactive or primary depression may aggravate disability and that patients may benefit greatly from supportive psychotherapy. Tricyclic antidepressants can be useful because of their combined anticholinergic and antidepressant effects.

Cranial-cervical Dystonia

Goals for physical treatment vary, based on the individual combination of dystonic movements and postures. Rehabilitation of tonic postures aims at providing balance between the action of individual muscles that control head position, while rehabilitation of rapid dystonic movements tends to provide motor control by replacing involuntary and inappropriate head movements with conscious and coordinated action. Specific exercises should aim toward avoiding abnormal secondary postures of the shoulders and trunk. The weeks following treatment with BoNT are the ideal time to carry out physical interventions, also taking advantage of progressive weakening induced by BoNT injections.

Supporting techniques include EMG biofeedback, visual control, and isometric exercise of contralateral muscles. Stretching and selective muscle strengthening are indicated when secondary alterations of neck muscles occur. Long-term neck muscle vibration (15 minutes) may provide transient relief in patients with cervical dystonia. Speech therapy may be useful in addition to BoNT treatment in spasmodic dysphonia cases.

Occupational and Upper Limb Dystonia

Physical treatment is indicated particularly in combination with splinting for occupational dystonia of the upper limbs. Immobilization is useful in association with BoNT treatment and rehabilitative treatment for severe focal occupational dystonia of the hand and forearm. Several issues need to be defined on larger series: the duration of splinting, the number of joints to

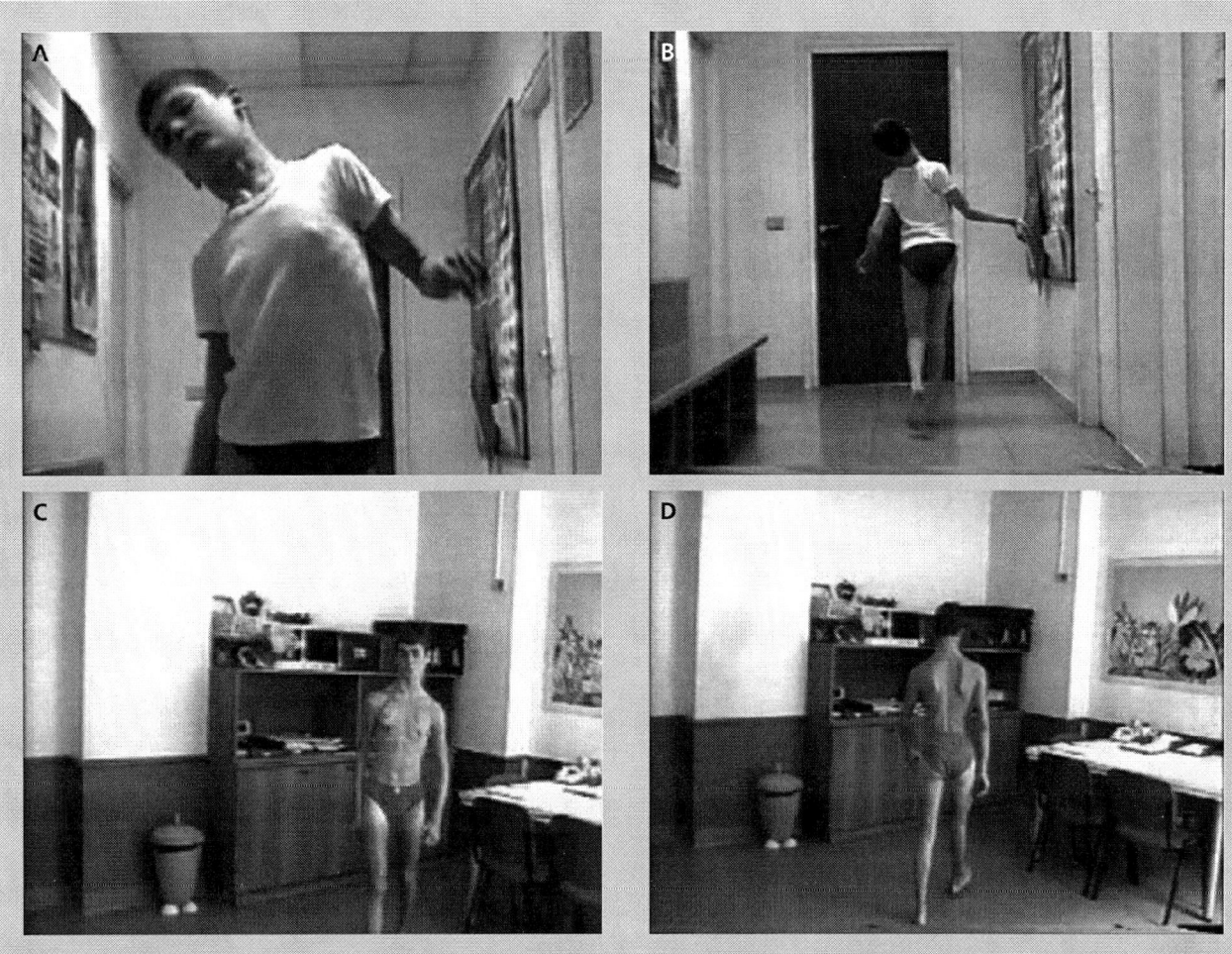

FIGURE 5.3 A patient with generalized dystonia and prominent axial involvement shown before (a, b) and 6 months after implant with high-frequency stimulation implant in the GPi (c, d). The improvement in posture and gait is evident from these still frames taken from video clips (courtesy of Dr. Nardocci).

splint, and the clinical features that could predict which patients are expected to benefit from immobilization.

Well-fitted braces are designed primarily to improve posture and to prevent contractures. Although children, in particular, may tolerate braces poorly, in some cases, these might be used as a substitute for sensory tricks. One concern about immobilization of a limb, particularly of a dystonic limb, is that such immobilization can actually increase the risk of exacerbating or even precipitating dystonia, as demonstrated in post-traumatic cases.

Specific rehabilitation programs have been designed for occupational dystonias and, particularly, for writer's cramp. From 6 to 18 months are needed to correct writer's cramp; stopping rehabilitation too soon can lead to a relapse.

Future Developments: Gene Silencing

The familial form of generalized dystonia linked to DYT1 is caused in the vast majority of cases by a 3-nucleotide deletion in the TOR1A (DYT1) gene. The mutant torsinA protein is thought to have a dominant-negative or dominant-toxic effect. Gene silencing can be obtained by RNA interference, i.e., by engineering a complementary RNA (c-RNA) that binds the mutant TOR1A messenger RNA (mRNA). This c-RNA, called *small interfering RNA* (siRNA), is capable of inducing in vitro a degradation of the mutant mRNA to which it is linked, thus silencing the expression of mutant torsinA protein.

This cellular mechanism is promising. Once adequate vectors become available, gene silencing could be used in presymptomatic patients, preventing disease manifestation. Moreover, as DYT1 dystonia is caused by neural dysfunction, with no evidence of neural degeneration, use in early symptomatic patients could prevent progression and even restore function. However, in vivo trials are needed to verify the delivery of siRNA in animals.

CONCLUSION

The treatment of dystonia has significantly progressed through the last 20 years. The discovery of BoNT has for the first time provided sizable improvements in patients, and the development of DBS has produced new expectations. The latter technique is currently under scrutiny for the various forms of dystonia. General medications have been tested repeatedly in primary dystonia, but have not provided significant advances in generalized forms. Still, the combination of these 3 different approaches can help in managing difficult cases.

A cost-effectiveness analysis is difficult to perform; different market brands and dosages of medications need to be considered. In addition, a significant variability among countries can occur. Oral therapy has by far the lowest cost of all treatment options.

The prices of BoNT vary quite significantly, not only among different countries, but also within a country. It is not uncommon to obtain bulk discounts for large users, resulting in lower prices when compared with the official national retail price. Moreover, annual costs for BoNT treatments can be reduced by treating several patients in a single session to completely use the dose of BoNT contained in each vial.

BoNT treatment is more expensive than traditional oral treatment, peripheral surgery, or physical therapy and supportive therapy alone (for example, casting). The additional costs for BoNT A treatment, however, often appear modest compared with the benefit provided to patients. In focal dystonia, and particularly in blepharospasm, BoNT is the only treatment that can significantly help patients. In cervical dystonia, the dose per patient can be up to 10-fold greater than that used in blepharospasm, while the duration and the clinical efficacy are lower. Finding the best trade-off between the amount of BoNT injected and clinical efficacy can improve cost-effectiveness.

Surgical procedures (including intrathecal baclofen, ablative surgery, DBS, and peripheral surgery) are more expensive than common oral therapy or BoNT, as they require hospitalization and operative costs, but with regard to generalized dystonia, in selected patients they can be more effective than standard medical treatments.

DBS is more expensive than ablative surgery performed on the same target, as it requires implanted material (leads, internal pulse generators, connectors). No cost-effectiveness analysis has been performed so far, because this therapy is quite recent and has been used in a relatively small number of patients. It should be considered that DBS involves high initial costs in the first year (especially when considering the possible temporary or permanent side effects). The cost of DBS is based directly on the cost of the device and the implant procedure. Thereafter, the cost per year decreases significantly, even when it becomes necessary to replace an exhausted internal pulse generator (usually 2 to 3 years after implant). DBS is considerably more expensive than common medical treatment when direct medical costs are considered in a short-term follow-up. In selected patients, however, DBS could produce a greater benefit (thereby becoming cost-effective). Improvement in self-care and activities of daily living reduces the necessity for caregivers and for supporting material. Monetary evaluation of these aspects is difficult and needs to be considered for an adequate follow-up period. So far, however, no studies are available for long-term efficacy and long-term side effects.

Genetic analysis provides a modern key to classification. There is no clear correspondence between available treatments and genetic classification, but it is expected that, in the near future, some genetically defined forms of dystonia will have specific treatment protocols.

ADDITIONAL READING

Bentivoglio AR, Albanese A. Botulinum toxin in motor disorders. *Curr Opin Neurol* 1999;12:447–456.

Brans JW, Lindeboom R, Snoek JW, Zwarts MJ, van Weerden TW, Brunt ER, et al. Botulinum toxin versus trihexyphenidyl in cervical dystonia: a prospective, randomized, double-blind controlled trial. *Neurology* 1996;46:1066–1072.

Brin MF. Treatment of dystonia. In: Jankovic J, Tolosa E, (eds.) *Parkinson's Disease and Movement Disorders*. Baltimore: Williams & Wilkins; 1998:553–578.

Burke RE, Fahn S, Marsden CD. Torsion dystonia: a double blind, prospective trial of high-dosage trihexyphenidil. *Neurology* 1986;36:160–164.

Jankovic J, Brin MF. Therapeutic uses of botulinum toxin. *N Engl J Med* 1991;324:1186–1194.

Lang AE. Surgical treatment of dystonia. *Adv Neurol* 1998;78:185–198.

Marsden CD, Marion MH, Quinn NP. The treatment of severe dystonia in children and adults. *J Neurol Neurosurg Psychiatry* 1984;47:1166–1173.

CHAPTER 6

REHABILITATION EXERCISES

Daniel Truong, MD, Mayank Pathak, MD, and Karen Frei, MD

SPECIFIC EXERCISES THAT CAN BE DONE AT HOME

This chapter describes some exercises that patients can perform on their own. The exercises are specific for the treatment of spasmodic torticollis (ST) and are designed to accomplish two major goals:

1. Stretch and relax the overactive agonist muscles that are in spasm.
2. Strengthen the antagonist muscles that can oppose the torticollis and bring the head position back to neutral.

The exercises in this chapter are designed to be used in conjunction with medical treatments such as oral medications, chemodenervation injections, physical therapy, and pain management interventions. In general, the stretching exercises will be applied to the overactive agonist muscles in conjunction with chemodenervation. As the overactive muscles are weakened by chemodenervation, they will be easier to stretch using the above exercises. As the agonists relax and their pulling force diminishes, it will become easier to perform strengthening exercises on the opposing antagonist muscles.

The particular exercises appropriate for a given patient will depend upon the muscles involved in that patient's particular case of ST. The treating physician should specify for the patient which muscles are acting as agonists, that is, those being injected with botulinum toxin (BoNT). The patient should practice those stretching exercises specific to the agonist muscles, along with exercises for any antagonist muscles the physician recommends for strengthening. In most cases, the antagonists will be those muscles that correspond to the agonists on the opposite side of the neck, but additional antagonists may need strengthening as well. A physical therapist can help the patient learn to perform the exercises properly.

The exercises have been designed to be performed with a bare minimum of easily obtained equipment. With a few modifications, they can be performed in almost any setting, at home or at work. All of the exercises described are to be performed slowly. If any movement produces pain, patients should be instructed that they should stop and seek further advice from their physician.

STRETCHING EXERCISES

The first exercises are simple stretches. Many of the following stretching exercises can be done in the standing or seated position. Most require some type of suitable handhold. In the standing position, the height of the handhold should be about the mid-thigh level, close to where the hand rests naturally. A suitable object to grasp might be a heavy table or desk. In the seated position, a sturdy chair with a suitable leg or crossbar should suffice. For some exercises requiring a handhold in front of the patient, the front edge of the seat may be grasped. A stable chair with a backrest and without wheels should be used. The figures depict a common type of inexpensive metal folding chair available at most office or home warehouse stores.

Exercise 1: Splenius Capitis, Levator Scapuli, and Others

This exercise is designed to stretch and relax the muscles that run down the back of the neck on either side of the neck bones, as well as the muscles that connect these bones to the shoulder blades. It may be useful for individuals who have a component of rotational torticollis plus retrocollis (as in Figure 6.1). It is performed in a seated position on a chair that allows the patient to grasp and hold on underneath. Alternatively, it can be performed in the standing position next to an object that has a handhold at approximately the mid-thigh level. Stretching for the left-sided muscles will be described. The entire procedure may be reversed if the patient requires stretching of the right-sided muscles.

The patient should grasp the handhold with the left hand, slowly lean the body forward and toward the right side, and at the same time allow the left shoulder to relax and be pulled downward while keeping a grip on the handhold. A pulling or stretching sensation

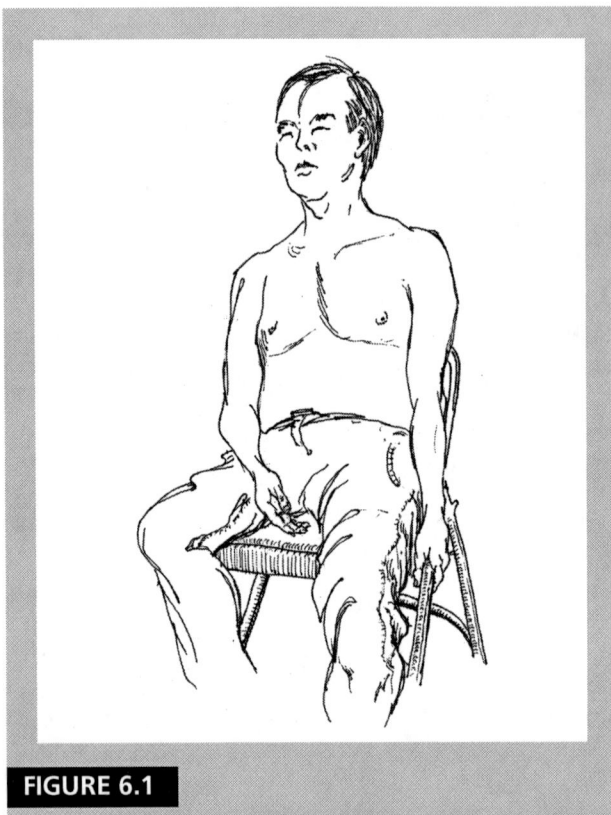

FIGURE 6.1

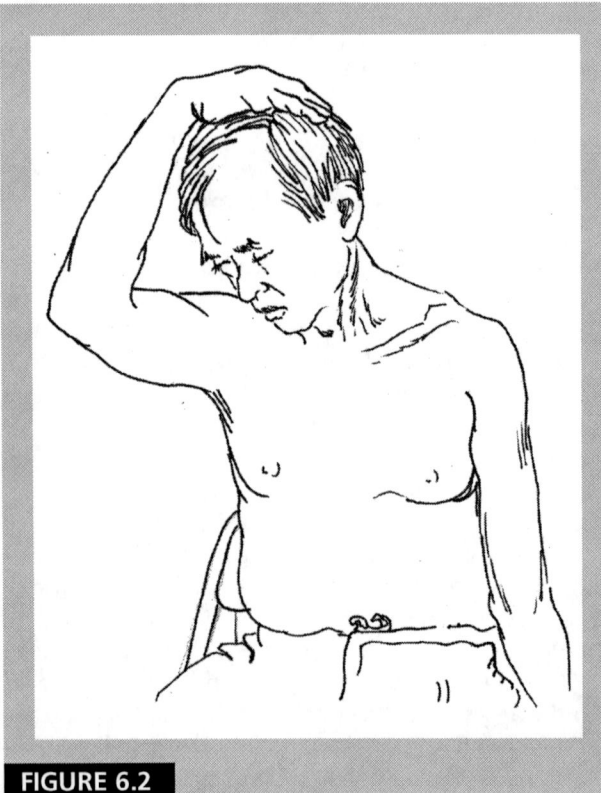

FIGURE 6.2

deep in the shoulder muscles may be felt. Next, the head is turned about 45° toward the right, then tilted into a direction away from the left arm. Doing this, the patient should feel the stretch in the muscles of the shoulder and the back of the neck on the left side. This position is held for 30 seconds. The sensation of stretch may then begin to subside, at which point the patient may actually be able to stretch a little further. To make the stretch even more effective, the patient should reach over the top of the head with the right hand and gently help pull along the direction of the stretch (Figure 6.2). This position should be held for another 10 seconds, than slowly released, followed by relaxation.

Exercise 2: Sternocleidomastoid on One Side

This exercise is intended to provide stretch to the sternocleidomastoid (SCM) muscle, which runs diagonally across the front and side of the neck and has attachments at the collar bone and the back of the skull. The SCM is one of the muscles most frequently involved in ST. The left SCM's normal action is to rotate the head toward the right while also tucking the chin downward to the chest. The movements in this particular exercise are somewhat complex, and require some patience and practice to be performed correctly. Stretching for the left SCM will be described. The entire procedure may be reversed if the patient requires stretching of the right SCM.

In order to stretch the left SCM, the patient begins in a seated or standing position and grasps the handhold behind or underneath with the left hand (Figure 6.3). The patient next leans the body slightly so that the left shoulder is pulled downward. By relaxing the shoulder, the patient will find that the collarbone is pulled downward. The head is now slowly rotated toward the left side (the side being stretched). Once the head has been rotated as far as it can comfortably go, the patient begins tilting it backward so that the chin moves toward the ceiling, then tilts the head slightly so that the right ear moves closer to the right shoulder (Figure 6.4). As this is done, the patient may feel a stretching sensation from the left collarbone to the side of the neck. The position should be held at the point of feeling stretch, but not pain. After 30 seconds, the feeling of stretch may begin to subside. At this point, the patient may increase the stretch a little further by cupping the fingers of the left hand around the chin and slowly and gently pushing upward. As always, the patient should stop if any pain is felt. This position should be held for 10 more seconds, then slowly released, followed by relaxation.

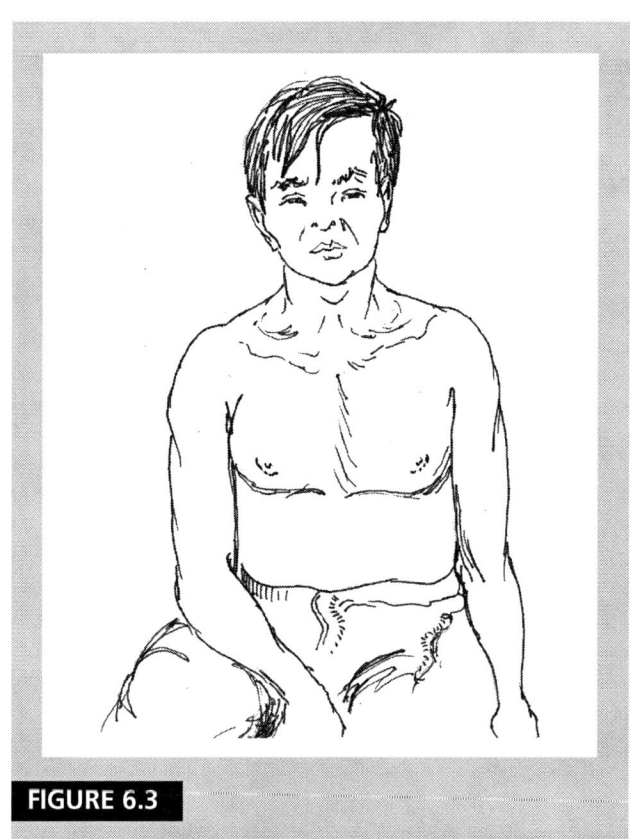

FIGURE 6.3

Exercise 3: Sternocleidomastoid on Both Sides

This exercise is a simple alternative stretch for the SCM that stretches both sides at once, and may be useful for individuals with anterocollis. This is best done in a seated position in a chair with some support for the back (Figure 6.5). The patient simply grasps a hand-hold behind or underneath with both hands, slowly leaning the body backward to pull down the shoulders. The shoulder muscles are allowed to relax, pulling down the collarbones. The head is kept in the neutral position facing directly ahead. Next the head is slowly tilted backward so that the chin moves toward the ceiling (Figure 6.6). The patient should feel a stretching sensation in the front and side of the neck. The shoulders should not be hunched up; they should be allowed to relax and be pulled downward, then held at the point where the stretch, but not unusual pain, is felt. This position should be held for 30 seconds, then slowly released, followed by relaxation.

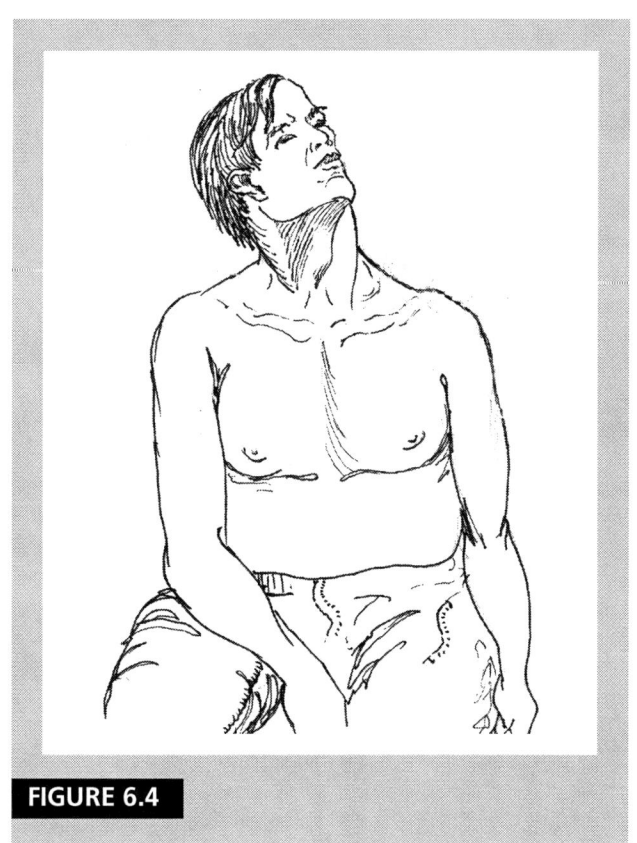

FIGURE 6.4

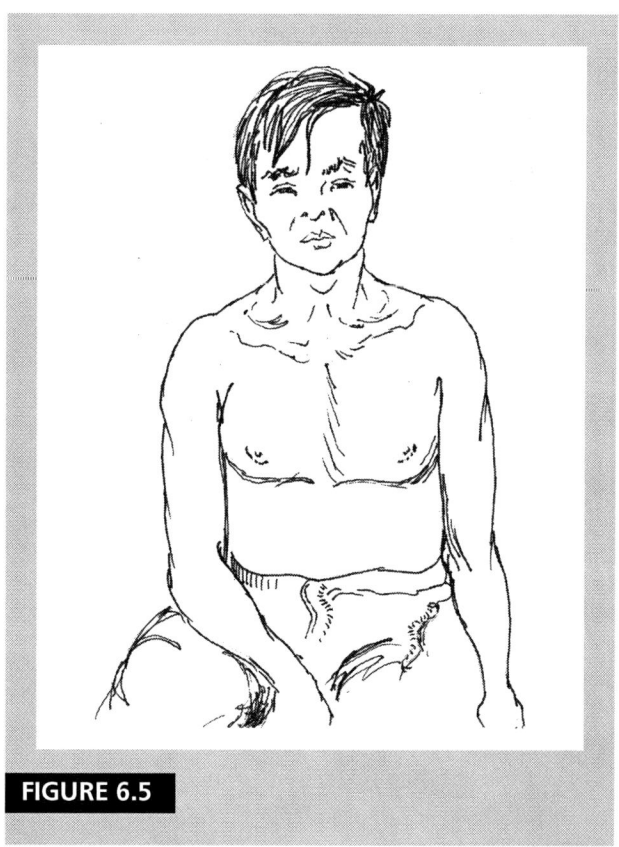

FIGURE 6.5

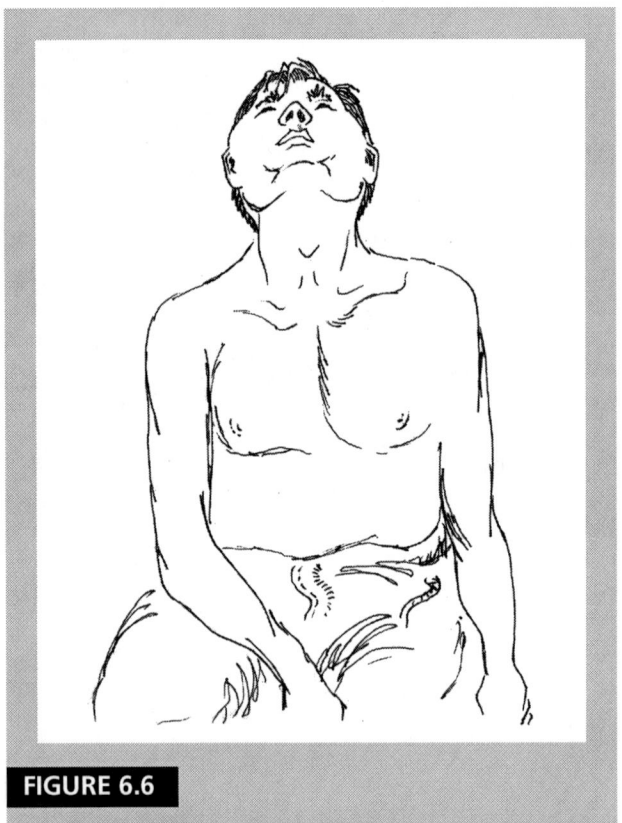

FIGURE 6.6

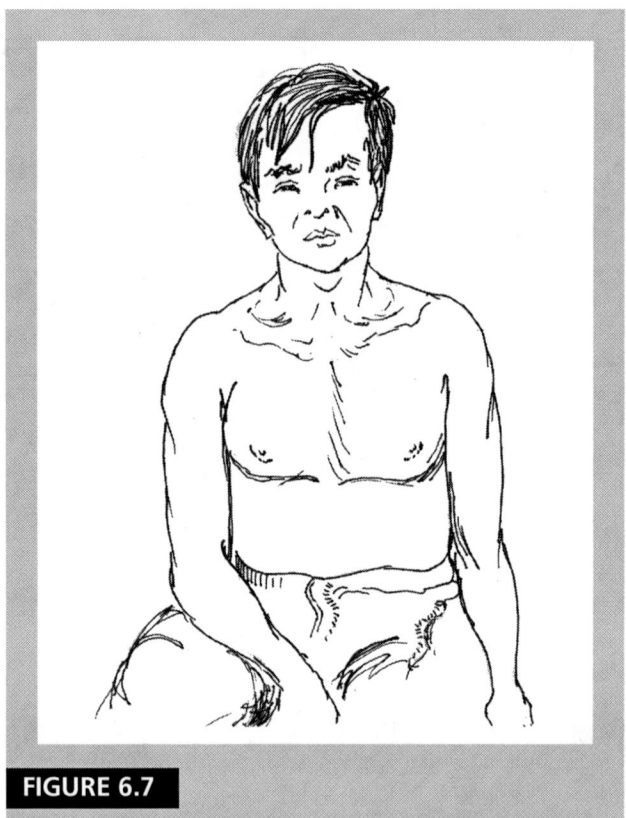

FIGURE 6.7

Exercise 4: Trapezius, Levator Scapuli, Sternocleidomastoid, and Scalenes

This exercise is intended to provide stretch for the muscles—mainly the trapezius and levator scapuli, but also the scalenes and sternocleidomastoid—that lift the shoulder upward and tilt the head directly sideways. This exercise is useful for persons who have lateralcollis. Stretching for the left-sided muscles will be described. The entire procedure may be reversed if the patient requires stretching of the right-sided muscles.

Starting from the seated or standing position, the patient grasps a handhold with the left hand (Figure 6.7), leaning the body to the right while relaxing the shoulder muscles and allowing the shoulder to be pulled downward. Next, the head is tilted sideways to the right. A stretching sensation from the shoulder to the side of the neck may be felt. This position should be held for 30 seconds. The sensation of stretching may begin to subside, at which point the patient can increase the stretch a little further by placing the right hand over the top of the head and slowly and gently pulling to the right (Figure 6.8). The stretch should be stopped if any unusual pain is felt. This position should be held for another 10 seconds, then slowly released, followed by relaxation.

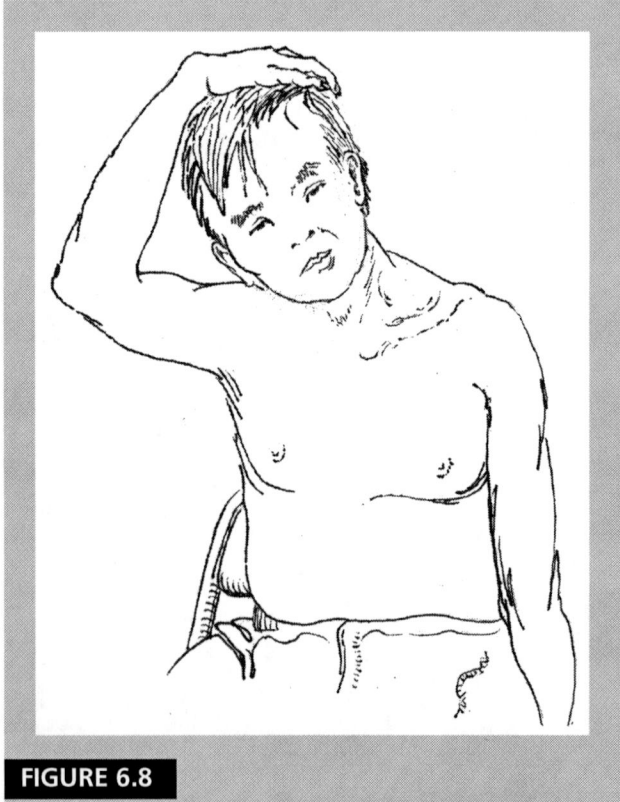

FIGURE 6.8

Exercise 5: Splenius Capitis

This exercise is intended to provide stretch to several muscles in the back of the neck, mainly the splenius capitis (SC), which starts at the neck bones and runs diagonally upward and outward to the base of the skull. The normal action of the right SC is to pull the head backward and rotate it slightly to the right side. This exercise is similar to exercise 1, but is more specific for the SC. Stretching for the right SC will be described. The entire procedure may be reversed if the patient requires stretching of the left SC.

To stretch the right SC, the patient starts in the seated or standing position, next rotating the head toward the left, then tilting it downward, tucking in the chin toward the chest (Figure 6.9). The patient may begin feeling a stretching sensation in the back of the neck, on one or both sides. This position should be held for 30 seconds. The stretching sensation may begin to subside, at which point the patient may increase the stretch a little further by placing the fingers against the side of the chin and gently pushing to rotate the chin toward the left shoulder (Figure 6.10). This position should be held for another 10 seconds, then slowly released, followed by relaxation.

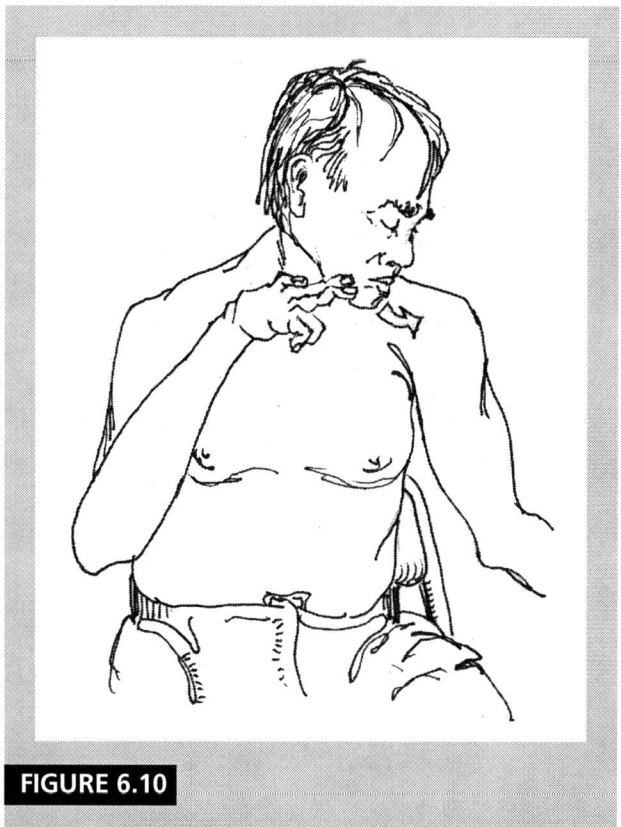

FIGURE 6.10

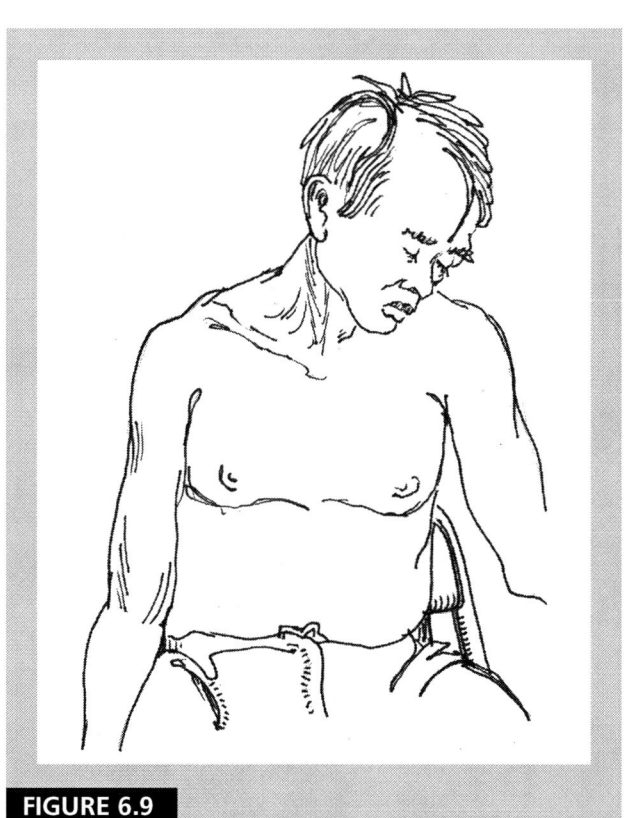

FIGURE 6.9

STRENGTHENING EXERCISES

The next set of exercises is designed to strengthen the antagonist muscles. Strengthening these muscles can help to bring the head back to the neutral position. To strengthen any muscle, it is necessary to use it to exert a force against resistance. Thus, to perform these exercises, a suitable object against which to push is needed. A pillow-sized block of soft foam rubber works best and may be obtained from a medical supply store or pharmacy. A larger, thick block of foam is best. Suitably thicker foam pillows may also be found in department and bedding stores. Most of the following exercises can be modified for performance in the sitting, standing, or lying position. In most cases, resistance supplied by an opposing hand or fingers can be substituted for the foam block or pillow, allowing the exercises to be performed in almost any situation. If the patient is not able to perform an exercise against resistance, the movement by itself should first be tried, using no type of resistance.

Exercise 6: Sternocleidomastoid on One Side

This exercise is designed to strengthen the SCM muscle on 1 side. Overactivity of the *right* SCM produces rotational torticollis toward the *left* (Figure 6.11), in which case strengthening of the *left* SCM is required.

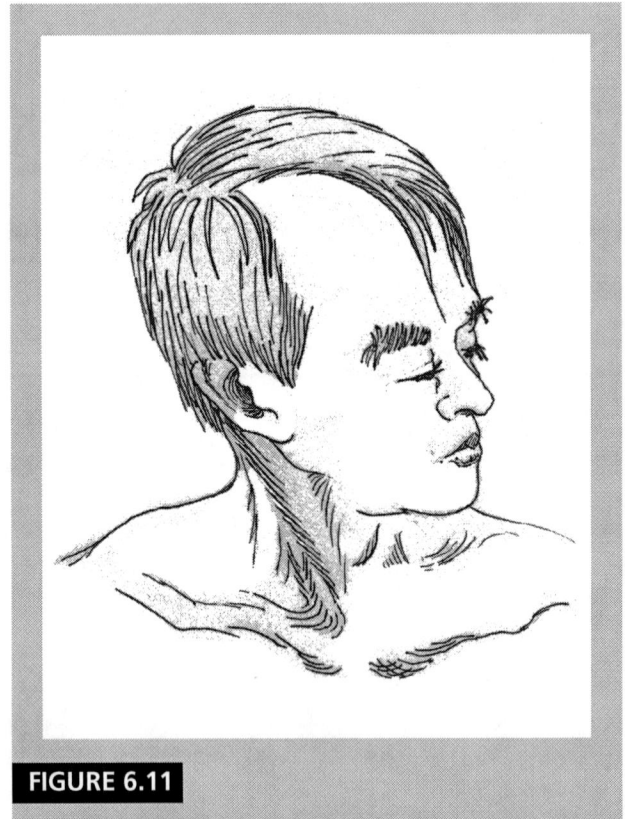

FIGURE 6.11

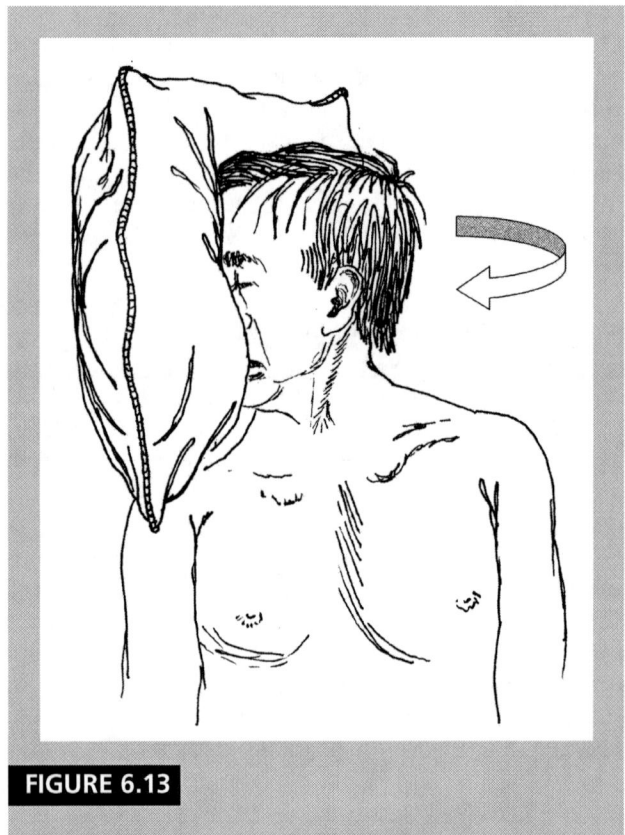

FIGURE 6.13

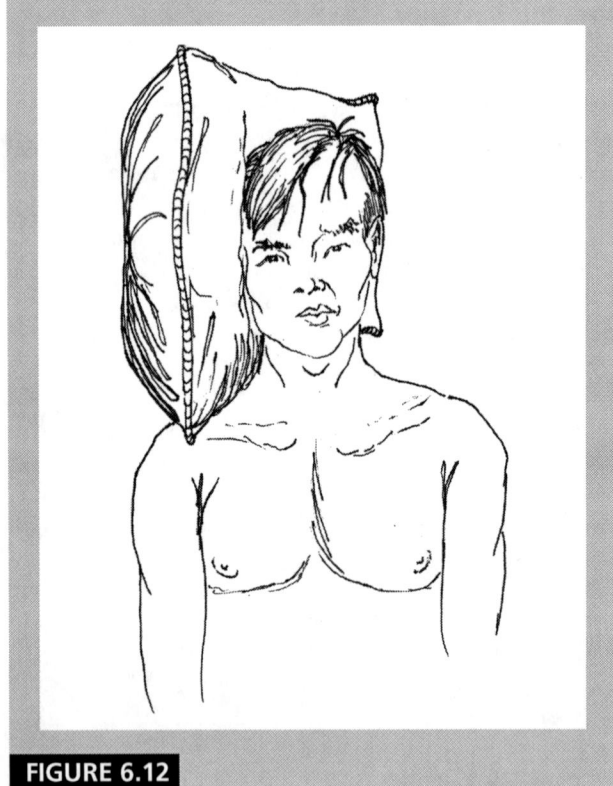

FIGURE 6.12

This entire procedure may be reversed if the patient requires strengthening of the right SCM.

To strengthen the left SCM, the patient starts in a seated position parallel to a wall. The right shoulder should just barely touch the wall. The foam block is placed on top of the right shoulder flush with the wall (Figure 6.12), with the side of the face placed snugly against the block. Next the head is turned slowly as if looking to the right, then rotated until it is pressing as hard as is comfortably possible (Figure 6.13). This position is held for 30 seconds, then released, and followed by relaxation. This exercise should be repeated 3 to 5 times per exercise session, and increased as tolerated. Some people may only be able to perform this exercise without a pillow; resistance provided by placing a hand on the side of the face may suffice. Others may not be able to push against a resistance at all.

Exercise 7: Trapezius and Levator Scapuli

This exercise is intended to strengthen the muscles that elevate the shoulder and shoulder blade, mainly the trapezius and the levator scapuli. Stretching the left-sided muscles will be described. The entire procedure may be reversed if the patient requires strengthening of the right-side muscles.

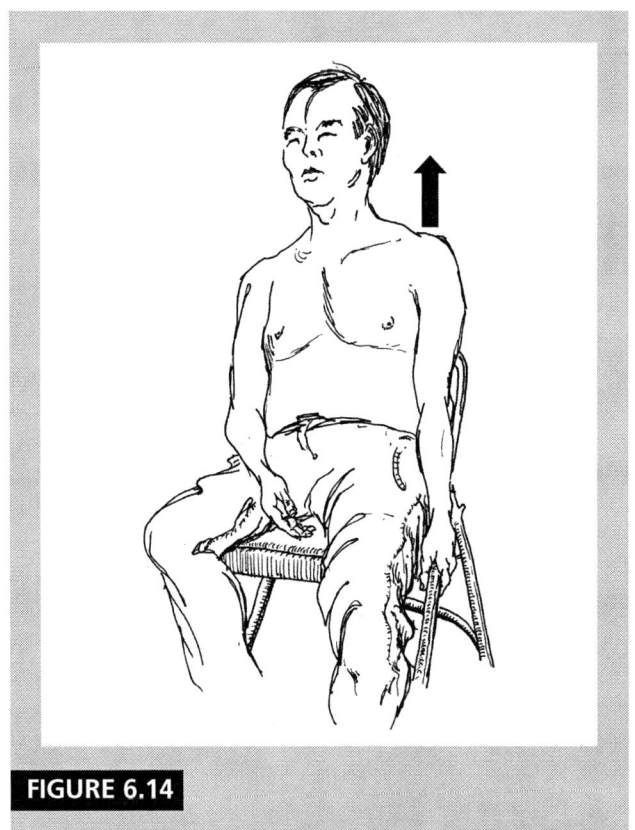

FIGURE 6.14

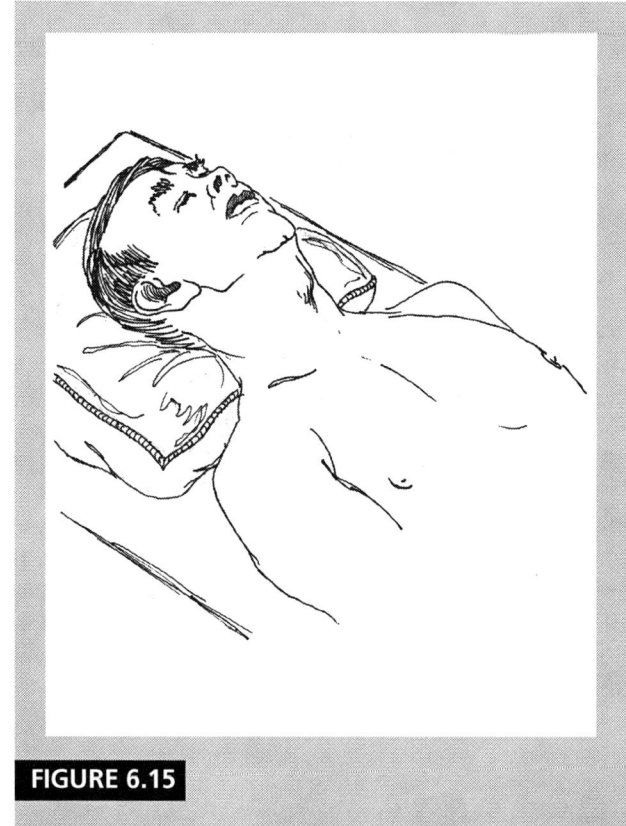

FIGURE 6.15

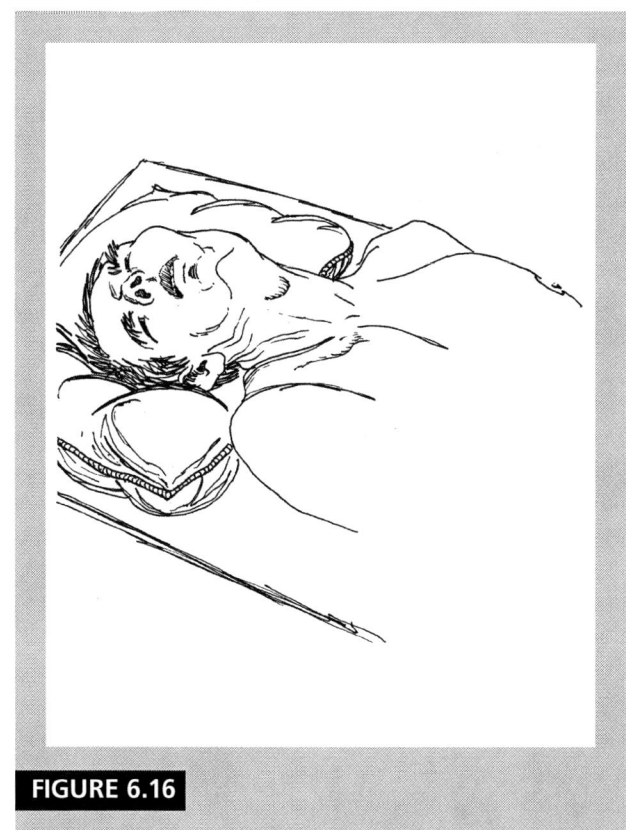

FIGURE 6.16

To strenthen the left-sided muscles, the patient starts in the seated or standing position and grasps a handhold with the left hand. The patient then slowly shrugs the left shoulder without moving the head (Figure 6.14). The pulling should be done with the shoulder shrug only. The patient should try to keep the arm straight and not try to lift by bending the arm at the elbow. The patient should pull with the shoulder muscles as hard as comfortably possible, hold for 30 seconds then slowly release and relax. This exercise should be repeated 3 to 5 times per exercise session, increasing as tolerated to a maximum of 12 repetitions.

Exercise 8: Splenius Capitis and Others on One Side

This exercise is designed to strengthen the muscles that lie along the back of the neck on either side of the neck bones. These include the diagonally running SC and other deeper muscles. The left SC tilts the head backward and turns the chin slightly toward the left. Strengthening of the right SC will be described. The entire procedure may be reversed if the patient requires strengthening of the left SC is depected in Figure 6.1.

To strengthen the right SC, the patient starts the exercise lying on the back with the foam pillow underneath the head (Figure 6.15), rotating the head approximately 45° to the right. The head is then tilted backward, pushing it into the foam pillow (Figure 6.16). The patient should try to push against the block with the part of the head immediately behind and above the right ear, pushing as hard as comfortably possible, hold for 10 seconds, then slowly release and relax. This exercise should be repeated 3 to 5 times per exercise session, increasing as tolerated, to a maximum of 12 repetitions.

Exercise 9: Sternocleidomastoids on Both Sides

This is an alternative exercise that can be used if both the right and left SCM muscles need to be strengthened. It may be useful for individuals with retrocollis. The patient starts by lying flat on the back (Figure 6.17), next lifting the head straight upward and tilting the chin slightly toward the chest. If desired, 2 fingers can be pushed against the forehead to provide resistance (Figure 6.18). This position should be held for 10 seconds, then slowly released. Relaxation should follow. The patient should repeat this exercise 3 to 5 times per exercise session, increasing as tolerated, to a maximum of 12 repetitions.

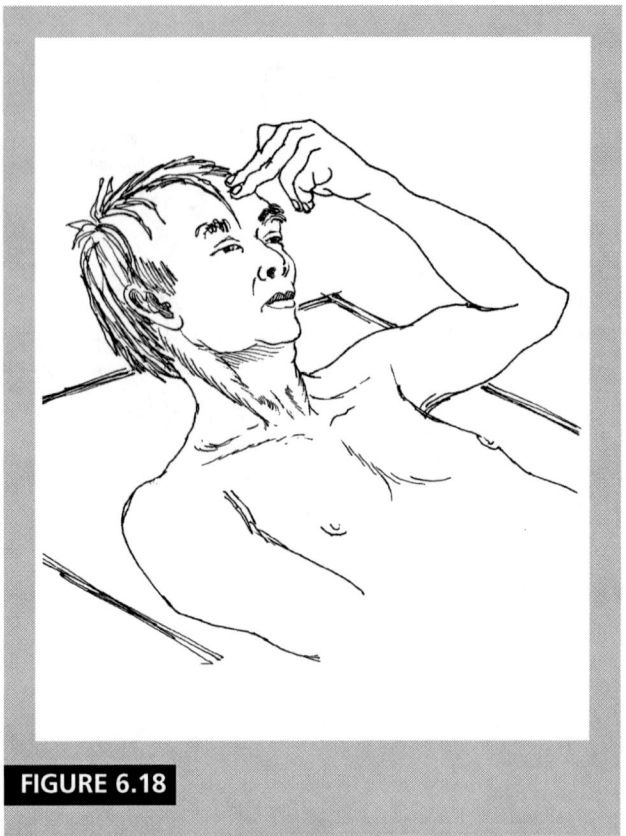

FIGURE 6.18

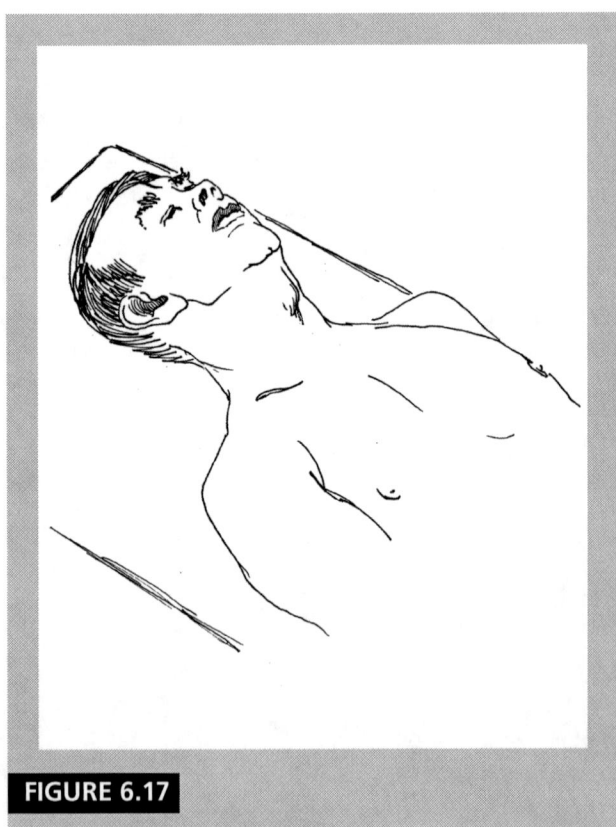

FIGURE 6.17

Exercise 10: Sternocleidomastoid, Trapezius, Levator Scapuli, and Scalenes

This exercise is designed to strengthen the muscles that tilt the head sideways and elevate the shoulder, including the SCM, trapezius, and levator scapuli. Strengthening for the right-sided muscles will be described. The entire procedure may be reversed if the patient requires strengthening of the left-sided muscles.

To strengthen the right-sided muscles, the patient begins in the seated position on a chair with the right shoulder touching the wall. The foam pillow is placed on top of the right shoulder flush with the wall, and the side of the head is placed snugly against the pillow (Figure 6.19). The head is next tilted directly sideways to the right, pushing into the foam pillow (Figure 6.20). The patient should push as hard as comfortably possible, holding for 10 seconds, then slowly release and relax. This exercise should be repeated 3 to 5 times per exercise session, increasing as tolerated, up to 12 repetitions. Some individuals may only be able to perform this exercise without a pillow; resistance provided by the hand against the side of the face may suffice. Others may only be able to perform the movement against no resistance at all.

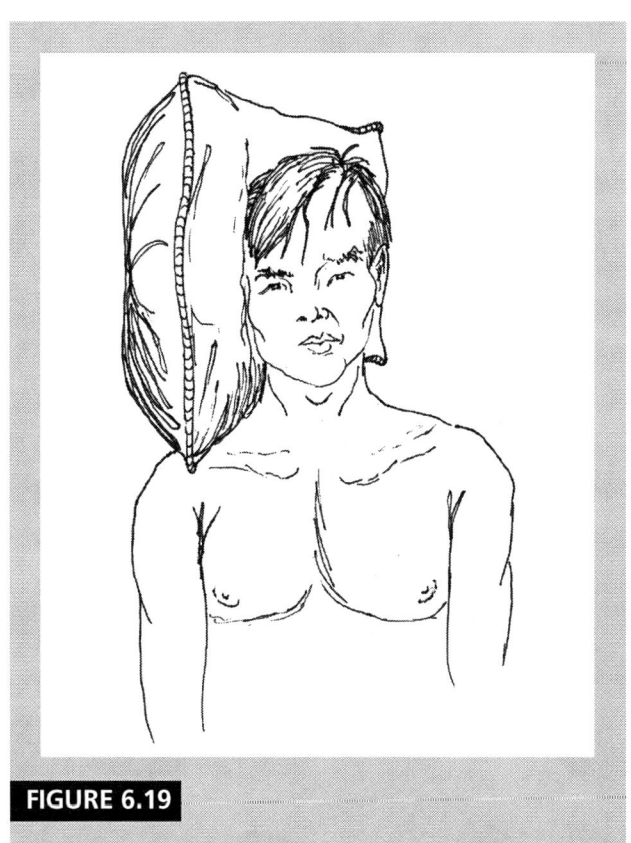

FIGURE 6.19

Exercise 11: Splenius Capitis and Others on Both Sides

This exercise is designed to strengthen all of the muscles that tilt the head straight backward. Including the SC, these lie along the back of the neck on either side of the spine. This exercise may be useful for people with anterocollis. The patient begins by lying on the back on a firm surface with the foam pillow underneath the head (Figure 6.21), then tilting the head straight backward, pushing into the foam block (Figure 6.22). The patient should push as hard as comfortably possible, hold for 10 seconds, then slowly release and relax. This exercise should be repeated 3 to 5 times per exercise session, increasing as tolerated up to 12 repetitions.

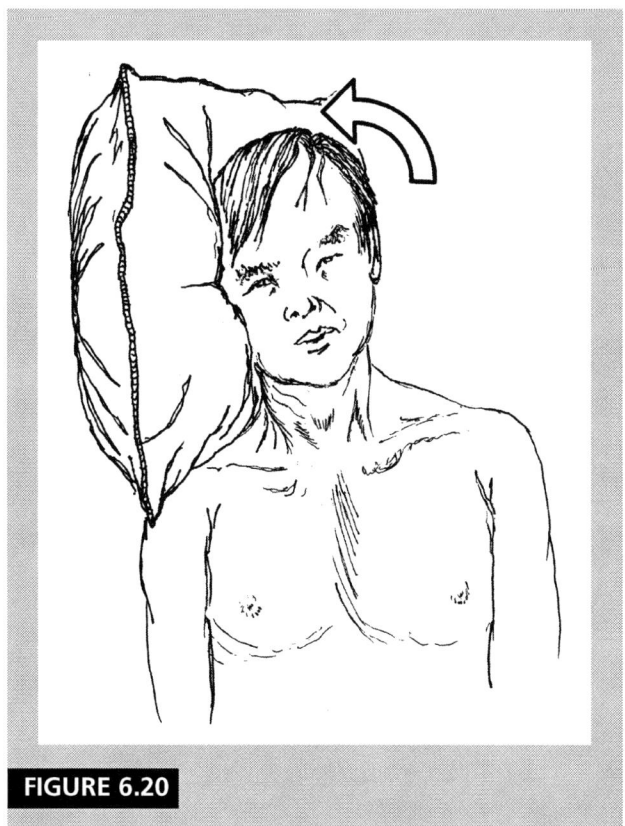

FIGURE 6.20

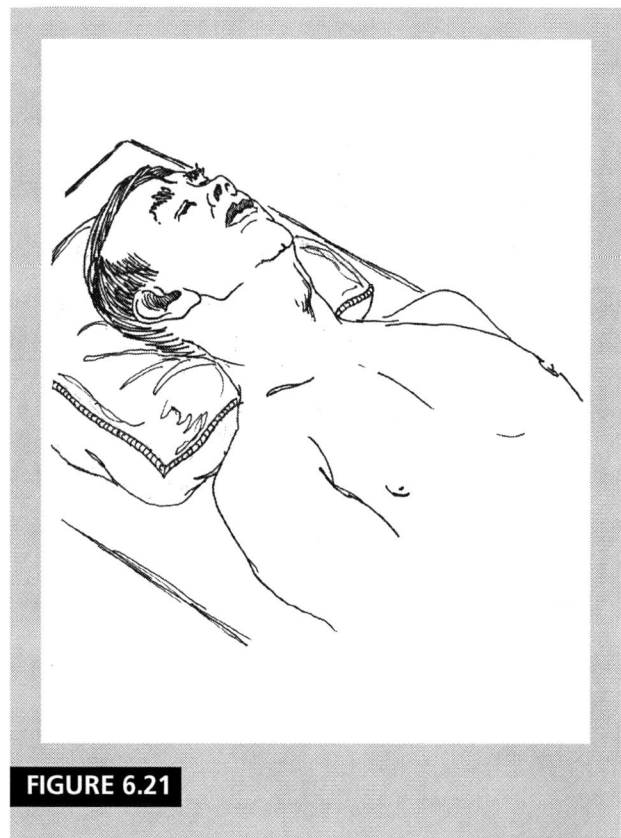

FIGURE 6.21

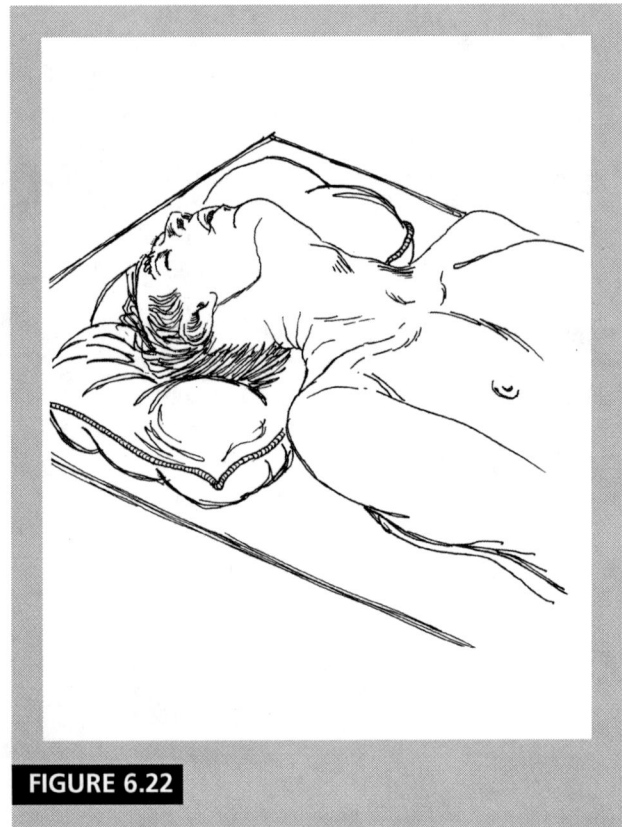

FIGURE 6.22

INDEX